STO

INSECTS & ALLERGY

by
**Claude A. Frazier, M.D.
and F. K. Brown**

INSECTS
and
ALLERGY

and what
to do
about them

University of Oklahoma Press : Norman

Other books on health by Claude A. Frazier, M.D.

Insect Allergy: Allergic and Toxic Reactions to Insects and Other Arthropods (St. Louis, 1969)

Should Doctors Play God? (editor) (Nashville, 1971)

Surgery and the Allergic Patient (editor) (Springfield, Ill., 1971)

Parents' Guide to Allergy in Children (New York, 1973)

Dentistry and the Allergic Patient (editor) (Springfield, Ill., 1973)

Games Doctors Play (editor) (Springfield, Ill., 1973)

Is It Moral to Modify Man? (editor) (Springfield, Ill., 1973)

Coping with Food Allergy (author) (New York, 1974)

Current Therapy of Allergy (editor) (Flushing, 1974; 2d. ed., 1978)

Doctor's Guide to Better Tennis and Health (editor) (New York, 1974)

Self-Assessment of Current Knowledge in Allergy (editor) (Flushing, 1976)

Psychosomatic Aspects of Allergy (New York, 1977)

Sniff, Sniff, Al-Er-Gee (St. Petersburg, Fla., 1978)

Insects and Allergy (with F. K. Brown) (Norman, 1980)

Library of Congress Cataloging in Publication Data

Frazier, Claude Albee, 1920–
    Insects and allergy and what to do about them.

    Bibliography: p.
    Includes index.
    1. Arthropoda, Poisonous—Venom—Toxicology.
2. Allergy. 3. Insect venom—Toxicology.
4. Insects. I. Franklin, Frieda Kenyon, 1921–
joint author. II. Title. [DNLM: 1. Insect bites
and stings. 2. Insects. 3. Hypersensitivity—
Etiology. WD430 F848ia]
RC598.A76F7   616.97   79-6706

We dedicate this book to
JOHN, JENNY, JULIE, and JEFF
and MR. and MRS. BELL

Contents

Contents

Contents

Illustrations

Preface

In the ground beneath our feet, in the air around us, in the water flowing down creeks and rivers to the blue craters of our lakes and the vast reaches of the seas, there is another, largely unnoticed world. Most of us are only vaguely and occasionally aware of its existence, yet it is a teeming, swarming, fiercely active world. I do not remember who made the head count or why, but it has been estimated that some 700,000 species inhabit this other part of our earthly kingdom, the realm of bug and beetle and bee.

We all belong to a kingdom, the kingdom Animalia. We human beings, however, are members of the phylum Chordata, while insects, as we generally call them, belong to the phylum Arthropoda. Arthropods are the "joint-foot" animals, and they have been amazingly successful down through the centuries, so much so that about 80 percent of the animal kingdom is made up of their various species. The two classes of arthropods that we will deal with in this book are the class Insecta, which includes bees, wasps, yellow jackets, fleas, ants, caterpillars, bedbugs, and lice; and the class Arachnida, which includes spiders, ticks, and scorpions. Since most of us lump all these together as insects, however, let us dispense with formality, as long as we understand that "insects" is our own lay terminology. It is not scientific, but it will facilitate our discussion. We are, after all, going to be more concerned with the medical and health aspects of the arthropods than we are with the creatures themselves, fascinating though they may be.

While there are many insects that we could cheerfully do without, the truth of the matter is that we could probably not survive if it were not for the existence of some of them. Such dependence may be mutual, although I am sure that there are some insects that would be just as happy if mankind disappeared from the scene. Man and insect have been on a collision course for thousands of years, and the former has done his level best to rid the kingdom of Animalia of as many of the latter as he could (not with any apparent success). The battle of the bug is not, however, the purpose of this book either. Rather I propose to deal with only two aspects of mankind's continual skirmish with insects—the health hazards posed by their stings, their bites, or their mere presence in the environment and what to do about those hazards. The book deals with those insects that commonly pose health problems in the United States. Each chapter is followed by a Reader's Guide that summarizes the main points of the chapter.

First, let us be aware of that presence. It has been estimated by an enterprising soul that about 425 million insects can comfortably inhabit a single acre of land. That sounds like standing room only, but of course some members of this huge phylum are so small as to be invisible to the unaided human eye. Unfortunately, even the tiniest of these mighty mites can cause trouble for human beings. Few of us can walk out into this teeming insect world unscathed. Some of us are exceptionally vulnerable to their assault. In fact, some of us are so sensitive to the venom of a single bee, for instance, that we can be "murdered" within ten to fifteen minutes.

Thus insects assume an importance in human health and welfare all out of proportion to their size.

INSECTS & ALLERGY

1

Insects: Friend and Foe

Insects are as fascinating as any little green men from Mars could possibly be. And much closer. They are tough: their propensity for survival has brought them down through approximately 250 million years. During the centuries that he has shared the earth with their many varieties, man has literally hunkered down on his heels to watch their meanderings, intrigued by their strange life cycles, their odd sex lives, their eerie depredations, their preferences in food, and the like. He has woven some wild tales about them, beginning somewhere back near the birth of Christ with Pliny's imaginings: giant ants of India that mined gold, butterflies that developed from the morning dew, bees that came from the head of a defunct ox. If you do not bury the head of the rattlesnake you kill, hornets will dine on it, and their venom will become as deadly as that of the snake itself. If you watch the daddy longlegs, he will tell you which way the cows went with a wave of one leg. The little green measuring worm moving with precise hitches up your sleeve is measuring you for a coffin. A cricket in the house will bring the family good luck.

Even today newspaper columns are devoted each fall to descriptions of caterpillars, especially the brown woolly bear. If his middle band is wide, the winter will be mild. Country folk go to the mud dauber to learn what nature intends for their crops: if the dauber builds his nest high, they say, the season will be wet; if low, near drought.

Insects even invade men's dreams. A dream about flies or bedbugs means that illness is on the way. A dream of bees swarming means death. And down in my country in North Carolina many people who keep bees will never sell them, although they will give them away, for they believe that selling bees will bring death to the buyer.

Not only are we fascinated by our tiny fellow travelers on the globe but also we share a love-hate relationship with them, and they with us. Not too many farmers, I suppose, would go along with the notion that insects in their fields are an asset. Fewer housewives would consider spiderwebs dangling from the ceiling an added attraction to the home. Yet actually, in spite of the immense amount of crop damage that insects cause and the diseases that they spread, some insects are mankind's allies in the battle for survival. The Bible illustrates our ambivalence toward them. On the one hand it speaks of a plague of grasshoppers and flies: "The land is as the Garden of Eden before them and behind them a desolate wilderness; yea, and nothing shall escape them" (Joel 2:3). Yet, on the other hand, it speaks approvingly of locusts and honey as "food fit for a feast."

This last is something we have been contemplating lately as we search desperately for sources of protein to fill the needs of our own too-fecund species. Some scientists declare that insects as food would provide more protein than beef, fewer calories than vegetables. And the housewife would be delighted at their probable price per pound. The house owner might be equally delighted to dispose of his termites fried in butter. Unlikely? Not in the least: termites are highly nutritious. In any case, various peoples have been eating insects all along. Close to home, Mexicans relish fried caterpillars, and our own southwestern Indians ate honey ants with pleasure. And there are always those delicious chocolate-covered ants on the novelty shelves of our markets. Scientists are experimenting around the world with the notion that insects are edible or that, at the very least, they can help us produce food.

In our own country one researcher has successfully raised housefly larvae on manure, then fed the larvae to chickens, who produced very good eggs and who themselves stayed very healthy. It may well be that in the near future the bane of our existence may become the bounty of a hungry world.

Even the much-feared killer bee, which we will discuss in Chapter 4, has her good side, for she produces about 50 percent more honey than her less aggressive cousin, the ordinary honeybee. Which, of course, explains why she got loose on our side of the world: African bees, brought to Brazil to be crossed with Brazilian honeybees to produce a superior honey maker, escaped their quarters, an event straight out of a monster-movie script.

Thus insects find their way to human tables as gourmet fare (and as not-so-gourmet fare accidently in such foods as cereals), and we eat the product of their labors. Moreover, without insects many of our crops would remain sterile, our fruit trees barren. Nature has seen fit to make the insect almost as essential to pollination as the wind. We will be very stupid and very hungry if we forget that.

There is more to say about the goody-goody side of the bug and the beetle and the bee. We have discovered fairly recently that insects can be used to control plant pests. For instance, when Klamath weed somehow was imported from Europe and spread across several million acres of California grazing lands, some intelligent soul turned to Europe for the leaf-eating beetle that throve on the weed in its native land. The beetle was delighted to oblige, and the spread of the weed was controlled. Fortunately, weed-eating insects are not catholic in their diet. They stick pretty much to a one-dish menu.

Nor are we human beings above turning insects against their own kind. Seed catalogs advertise praying-mantis egg cases and pints of ladybugs to help the gardener control vegetable and flower killers. Wasps that depend on other insects do a great service for mankind. Yellow jackets and Polistes wasps, for example, dine on the extremely destructive corn earworm and the armyworm. One kind of small wasp busies itself laying eggs in aphids. An aphid so chosen goes about its business for about three days and then begins to wither upon the vine, so to speak, as the wasp larva develops at the expense of the aphid's internal organs. There is even a horseguard wasp that flies about livestock catching horseflies and stable flies. (It is a little off our path here, but some of the parasitic wasps will lay one or more eggs within a caterpillar or other insect, and a number of offspring will develop from each egg. The poor host insect suddenly becomes "loaded." Needless to say, the load is lethel. Some insect species employ this strange method of reproduction to produce several thousand offspring from a single egg.)

So, as is ever the way, we must temper our curses against the malevolence of some insects with praises for those that are beneficial, at least for us.

Before we turn to the malevolent, we should note that there is one other, very odd way that insects are helpful. There is such a thing as a museum bug, actually akin to the carpet, or buffalo, beetle, whose larvae, when placed in a "bug room" along with the carcass of an animal wanted for an exhibit or study, nibble the bones clean as a whistle. There are two difficulties attached to the employment of this bug. One is that, if it gets loose in the museum itself, it can play havoc with the exhibits of stuffed birds, animals, and insects. The second problem is that certain spiders love to dine on the larvae and have a way of getting into the bug room and cleaning out the helpers.

I suppose that most of us consider insects to be scourges and believe that we could survive very nicely without them. It is sobering to realize that in our famine-stricken world millions of tons of food are destroyed annually by the depredations of insects. The World Health Organization has estimated that more than thirty-three million tons of bread grains and rice are lost each year. In the United States alone one-tenth of our commercial crops never leave the field, and every home gardener knows he must tithe to the bugs and the beetles:

One seed for the maggot, one for the crow.
One seed for the cutworm, and one to grow!

Insects: Friend and Foe

We have tried very hard to rid ourselves of a goodly number of insect pests that threaten our wherewithal, almost poisoning ourselves in the process. In fact, some of the insecticides that we have used in quantity have come uncomfortably close to taking us right out of the picture along with our targets. We still do not know what eventual effect some of the chemicals may have upon human health and future generations. Perhaps if we revive the dietary delights of locusts and honey, we will kill two bugs with one stone.

Apart from the general havoc that they have wreaked upon man's attempts to feed and clothe himself, insects have been a mighty hazard to human health, indirectly as disease vectors and directly through their own toxicity. As disease vectors they have often come very close to ridding the world of the human species. Fleas riding on the backs of rats almost halved the population of Europe during the plagues, and the louse took a heavy toll of both military and civilian populations during many of man's endless wars upon himself. The louse, in fact, often proved the more efficient killer as it delivered typhus and other dreaded diseases with strict impartiality to both sides in human conflicts. Even now it is estimated that 100 million people annually are stricken with malaria, thanks to the mosquito, and that about 800,000 die each year from the disease, mostly children under five. In West Africa especially, hundreds of thousands of people are robbed of their sight by a small black fly that carries a disease that they call river blindness and physicians call onchocerciasis. Africa is also the home of the tsetse fly, which carries sleeping sickness to people and their cattle.

We tend to belittle the power of bugs. Obviously it would behoove us to know them better.

They are small, yes, sometimes even microscopic, but smallness` seems to have been as asset in their survival. Another asset in their success down through the centuries probably has been the dominance of the female—a suggestion anti-women's-libbers might want to consider. The female is the be-all and end-all of the insect world. The male's role is brief—if he even exists. Many species simply reproduce without fertilization. Aphids, whose numbers can multiply with astonishing speed, are an example.

Insects may appear to us to be brainless since their brains are so tiny. That is not always the case, however. The minute brain of a bee, for instance, is probably the most highly organized bit of tissue to be found among living things. It may hold the bee to a rigid pattern of behavior and may not provide her the power to reason or remember, but it has ensured the survival of beedom for a long time. As far as we know, the brains of bees and beetles and other bugs do not envision blowing up the world. Thus our much-vaunted type of brain may not have as much survival value as we tend to think it has. The brain of an arthropod is actually a cerebral ganglion, within which is concentrated more nerve tissue than is found in the ganglia of the arthropod's segmented body. While each segment of the arthropod's body has its own controlling pair of ganglia, and these are almost autonomous, the head, or cerebral, ganglion accommodates the large number of sense organs and head appendages. In this sense it is a brain.

If insects' brains are small, their strength is not, for insects posses astonishing brawn for their size. An ant has been known to lift a weight fifty-two times that of its own tiny carcass. A man would have to hoist eight thousand pounds to achieve the same feat. A bee has been known to pull three hundred times its weight. A man would have to tow three trailer trucks hitched bumper to bumper down the highway to match that kind of power. A flea, though difficult for us even to spot, can broad jump what would be for a human being the equivalent of 700 feet and high jump over the equivalent of a 450-foot building. Just to keep a proper perspective on our own place in the scheme of things, we need to remind ourselves that brain size and body size are no indicators of a living thing's ability to survive. Nor is brain size any indicator of the harm a creature can inflict.

Aside from their role as disease vectors, insects can kill directly. In fact, they are responsible for more fatalities in our country each year than are poisonous snakes. Which is strange when one considers the fear and loathing that so many of us have for reptiles, as though we instinctively sense that they can be a threat. We tend to disparage insects, brushing them aside as more a nuisance than anything else. Many a snake gets battered to death for no other reason than that he is a snake; he dies because we fear him. On the other hand, we usually squash insects more out of loathing than out of fear.

An insect can kill in two ways: through injecting highly toxic venom with its bite or sting and through a victim's unusual susceptibility either to the venom or to other substances that the insect injects during its attack. The toxic reaction depends directly on the amount of venom injected, and fatalities are usually the result of multiple bites or stings. It has been estimated, for instance, that five hundred to eight hundred bee stings suffered within a short space of time can be lethal. There are cases on record, however, of individuals who have sustained many more stings than that and survived. There is an account, for instance, of a European in Africa who was attacked by a swarm of bees as he walked along a riverbank. The unfortunate man jumped into the shallow river as the bees literally coated his body from the waist up in what a report described as "a layer about three inches deep." As the bees stung him, the victim said later, "I felt an intense burning sensation as though I were on fire." As he tried to fight off the bees, he began to sicken from the effects of the venom. Vomiting, he managed to move into deeper water, where he sat down to try to protect his head with his shorts, receiving many more stings on his arms. He then tried to plaster himself with mud. He finally coated himself and his shorts thickly enough to keep the bees from stinging through the muck, but he still had to leave an air hole to breathe. The bees found it quickly and flew in to sting his face repeatedly. Finally, he resorted to biting them.

By now he was really a sick man. His head ached badly. He suffered from diarrhea so intense that he was incontinent and from "a continuous burning pain in his stomach." In the end that rugged but unfortunate man spent four and a half hours in the river.

When he finally was rescued and received medical attention, it was discovered that he had been stung 2,243 times. His face, neck, scalp, and body from the waist up were black with stings. Dead bees were matted in his hair. Doctors removed 221 stingers from his lips, his tongue, the interior of his mouth, and his eyelids. Miraculously he recovered after five days spent in the hospital.

In contrast to such toxic reactions as this, the reaction of an individual hypersensitive to insects depends less upon the volume of the venom or other substances injected and more upon the individual's own vulnerability. Hypersensitive individuals are allergic, and some are so much so that the sting of a single bee can send them into shock and even kill them within ten to fifteen minutes or less. For example, in the area of my native Asheville, North Carolina, not long ago a young man fishing one of the clear mountain trout streams was stung once or twice by either bees or yellow jackets. Almost at once he began gasping for breath. His face turned bluish gray as he became cyanotic, trying unsuccessfully to draw oxygen into his lungs. His companion tried to help him, but there was nothing he could do. Even if he had comprehended what was happening, he had no means to aid his friend. Within ten minutes the unfortunate young man was dead.

The insects dangerous to human beings in the United States are relatively few compared to other parts of the world, such as the tropics. Members of the Hymenoptera clan— honeybees, bumblebees, yellow jackets, wasps, hornets, and fire ants—sting and are to be avoided by the allergic and nonallergic alike. The scorpion is potently venomous. The black-widow and brown-recluse spiders are only a bit less so. Some sensitive individuals react strongly to the bites of various flies, such as deerflies and blackflies, and of mosquitoes. While most insect bites are not dangerous, they can cause a great deal of discomfort and make a shambles of the human skin. Fleas and mites, for instance, can raise bumps and cause intense itching on anyone, and other less common insects, such as wheelbugs, kissing bugs, blister beetles, and caterpillars, can hurt. It is as transmitters of disease, however, that insects have created the greatest problem for man. Millions of human beings have died from the disease that insects have spread. There have even been cases of plague in the United States during the last few years.

Before we go on to discuss the various arthropods and their impact on our health, we should first understand something about allergy and why the hypersensitive are in danger whenever they venture into the outdoor world unless they take proper steps to immunize and protect themselves.

By now the reader surely agrees that we cannot lightly dismiss the small but potent. Like Tonto and the Lone Ranger, we are surrounded. While we can tolerate the teeming insect populations up to a point, some among us must treat certain insect species as though they were the gruesome monsters of a late late TV show. Nevertheless, with proper knowledge of treatment, prevention, and management measures, the allergic and the nonallergic need not be unduly anxious. Cautious perhaps, but not afraid.

READER'S GUIDE: WHICH INSECTS BITE? WHICH STING?

Class Insecta—head, thorax, abdomen, 2 antennae, 4 wings, 6 legs.

HYMENOPTERA—typically 4 membranous wings, female usually has stinger in tail.

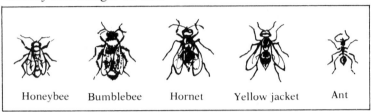

| Honeybee | Bumblebee | Hornet | Yellow jacket | Ant |

DIPTERA—2 membranous wings, 2 vestigial wings.

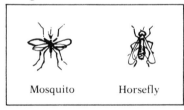

| Mosquito | Horsefly |

HEMIPTERA—winged or wingless, oval flattened body.

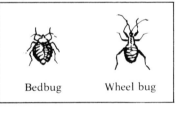

| Bedbug | Wheel bug |

COLEOPTERA—4 wings, one pair thickened

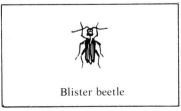

Blister beetle

SIPHONAPTERA—wingless, body compressed laterally, hind legs longer.

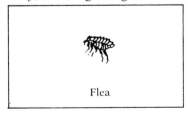

Flea

Insects: Friend and Foe

Class Arachnida—cephalothorax and abdomen, no antennae, 8 legs (adults).

ARANEAE—cephalothorax constricted from unsegmented abdomen, 6 organs for spinning webs.

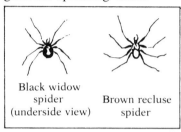

Black widow spider (underside view)   Brown recluse spider

ACARI—cephalothorax and abdomen united, many variations.

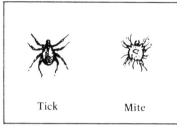

Tick   Mite

SCORPIONES—long body, segmented abdomen, narrow tail with poison stinger

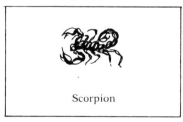

Scorpion

THE BITERS:
ant, mosquito, horsefly, bedbug, wheel bug, blister beetle, flea, spider, tick, mite.

THE STINGERS:
honeybee, bumblebee, hornet, yellow jacket, scorpion.

2

Unhappily
for Some . . .

Mr. J, recently retired, came from the city to the country with
a trunkful of ideals and idylls. His two-acre "ranch" was to be
a veritable Garden of Eden, complete with flowers, vegetable
garden, and fruit trees. Alas, there was to be a fly in the ointment, so to speak. Or rather a bee. Along with his dreams, Mr.
J brought city ignorance to the country. He had no concept
whatever of the world of insects that already inhabited his
acres, their squatter's rights well established. It was not long
before he ran afoul of a bunch of honeybees intent on gathering pollen and nectar from his newly planted flower beds and
blooming fruit trees. He was stung three times on the left
hand and arm.

Mr. J's outrage was immediate. What had he done to be so
set upon? What is more important to our intent here is that
his left hand and arm began to swell to alarming proportions.
From hand to shoulder the limb doubled in size. Mr. J's outrage turned to mild surprise. Mrs. J bustled a bit, tch-tch-ed,
and applied the old-fashioned remedy of baking soda to the
sting sites to lessen the initial pain and subsequent itching.
For the swelling she gave him ice packs. Aloud she wondered
whether going to see the doctor might not be a good idea.

Very sensible of her it was too. But Mr. J was too manly to
accept the good advice. In any case the swelling rapidly di-

14

minished, and only the itching persisted a day or two to remind him that he had been villainously attacked. Neither Mr. or Mrs. J was aware that such a swelling is a warning of possibly dire future consequences. Mr. J all but forgot about the incident and returned happily to his garden. He was a little wiser, of course, and far more wary of bugs that buzzed among his blossoms. But unhappily, before the summer was out, he was stung again, this time only once and on the side of the neck as he brushed past a bee-laden rose.

"Drat!"

He swatted wildly at his neck, but the damage was done. The bee wobbled off to die, leaving her abdomen, stinger, and venom sac—the latter still pulsing—in Mr. J's flesh. He started for the house, thinking of baking soda and an ice pack. Suddenly, however, he began feeling queer. His eyes began itching. He coughed, feeling constraint in his throat and chest. His heart began pounding, and he began sweating profusely. Red wheals broke out on his cheeks and arms. It became increasingly difficult to breathe. He was halfway to the house, feeling worse by the minute, when his knees gave way, and he sank to the ground unconscious.

Fortunately, Mrs. J who was trimming a box hedge nearby, had turned when she heard him mutter, "Drat!" Puzzled, she watched him swat at his neck, then start toward the house. When he collapsed, she dropped her shears and rushed to his side, fearing that he had had a heart attack.

Within twenty minutes Mr. J was in the emergency room of the local hospital. He was scarcely breathing. Heroic measures were taken to save his life. Emergency personnel assumed that they were dealing with a heart-attack victim, but as Mr. J returned slowly from the dim world of unconsciousness, he began muttering, "Damn bee," and rubbing at the side of his neck.

Resident physician, intern, and nurse all bent over him and looked again. There it was, stinger still embedded, tiny venom sac still attached. They knew then that they were dealing not with a heart attack but rather with a generalized systemic reaction, an allergic reaction, to bee venom. Mr. J had suffered anaphylactic shock and had come very close to dying. All because of a single bee sting.

Why?

Because Mr. J was allergic, severely allergic to honeybee venom.

Allergic? What is allergy anyway? What does "being allergic" mean? Well, a generally accepted definition of allergy is that it is an abnormal reaction to substances most people tolerate without problems. For instance, most of us can walk abroad through autumn fields abloom with ragweed and never even know it is there. Ragweed pollen does not raise so much as a sniffle or a sneeze. But a person allergic to ragweed need not even get close to the stuff to recognize that its pollen is adrift on the wind. The onset of hay fever informs him that the ragweed season has begun. Between 20 and 25 percent of the population, it is estimated, will be allergic to something at some time in their lives. Which is an awful lot of allergy!

That still leaves a lot to be explained.

Let me attempt to make a complex business somewhat simpler, but first you must know that allergy is not yet thoroughly understood, even by those who have practiced and researched in the field for many years. It is still one of those concepts that defy reduction to simplicity, like Einstein's theory of relativity.

An allergic reaction is really an immune reaction, a reaction against substances that the body recognizes as foreign. All of us, except for the occasional rare individual, possess immune systems that battle against the intrusion of substances harmful to our bodies. Some of us, however, possess immune systems that battle against harmless substances as well. Antibodies are our defense mechanisms, and we manufacture different groups of these antibodies, or immunoglobulins as they are called. Immunoglobulin E, mercifully shortened to IgE in the literature of allergy, is the antibody most closely associated with allergy diseases. We all possess some IgE as part of our immune systems, but the allergic individual appears to possess a greater quantity than the nonallergic person. For reasons not thoroughly understood, the allergic individual manufactures an overabundance of these particular antibodies. We believe that to some extent this is an inherited tendency. Statistically, if allergy runs in one side of a person's family, he has about a 50 percent chance of becoming allergic to something during his lifetime. If allergy runs in both sides of his family, his chances of being allergic increase to about 75 percent. He does not necessarily inherit the tendency to be allergic to the same substances as his forebears, however, or to register his allergy within the same body systems. For instance, a mother may be allergic to eggs and exhibit that sensitivity through her skin as eczema, whereas her son may be allergic to ragweed and exhibit his sensitivity through his respiratory system as asthma.

What causes the symptoms of allergy such as eczema or asthma?

Allergens (substances most likely to cause reactions in the sensitive individual) can be ingested, inhaled, or contacted by the individual or injected into him. The clash within the body as IgE antibodies meet allergens releases substances that are generally called chemical mediators. One such substance is histamine. The chemical mediators in turn cause the actual damage to the body tissues. IgE entibodies are bound to certain white blood cells and to mast cells, which are especially abundant in such organs as the smooth muscles (particularly those of the respiratory and gastrointestinal systems), the mucous glands, the mucous membranes, and the skin. Thus when an allergen such as bee venom arrives on the scene where IgE antibodies are in abundance, those tissues become a virtual battleground. Histamine, for instance, when released can cause the smooth muscles that are wrapped around the bronchi to constrict, thus narrowing the airways. That is why Mr. J suffered breathing difficulties during his reaction to the beesting.

That is not the whole story, though. The allergic individual may possess a tendency to react to allergenic substances with various symptoms, but he must first be sensitized to those substances. He must, so to speak, be set up for reaction. The first contact with allergens results in either no reaction or a "normal" reaction—the kind that most of us would have—although in the allergic individual the normal reaction may be more marked than for most people. Thus the first stings Mr. J suffered sensitized him to bee venom; he was "set up." Sometimes a patient who has had a bad reaction to an insect sting claims that it "came out of the blue," that he had never been stung before. Of course, he may have been stung in childhood and have long since forgotten it. But it is also possible that he is correct, for one can be sensitized by insect debris in the air, in water, and even in food. This is a somewhat esoteric subject, which I will later discuss in Chapter 21. Suffice it to note here that some individuals react with allergy symptoms to tiny bits of insect scales, wings, fecal matter, and the like that float in the air or that they swallow in food or water. With billions of insects busy in the immediate environment, the individual who is allergic to them in any form has a hard time of it. It has been estimated that about 17 percent of the population suffers from such an allergy. I believe that this figure may be a bit high, but it has been established that out of one thousand people four to eight have suffered or will suffer a generalized systemic reaction to insect stings or bites. These people are endangered, for a systemic reaction can be severe. It can even be fatal.

As with other types of allergies a number of factors affect the individual's sensitivity to insects. Usually, but not always, the amount of exposure is one such factor. Naturally, the more venom injected, the more allergenic saliva that is absorbed from a bite, the more chance there is of reaction. As we have noted, however, the severely allergic may react violently to the sting of a single bee or the bite of a lone deerfly.

Naturally, too, the potency of the allergen also plays a role in reaction. For instance, in the early spring and late fall the honeybee has far less venom in its venom sac than it has during the height of summer; and the potency of insect venom, of course, varies in different species.

The general health of the victim may also be a factor in the severity of his reaction, although it may not determine whether or not he is allergic. Some fatalities from insect stings have undoubtedly occurred because of underlying health conditions such as heart disease, but in most fatalities caused by anaphylactic shock (the severest form of generalized systemic reaction) health is not the main factor. We should also note that, in one study, over half the patients suffering allergic reactions to insect stings or bites exhibited other allergic conditions, such as hay fever, eczema, or asthma. Unhappily, it is often thus for allergic persons: if they are allergic to one thing, they tend to be allergic to something else. Thus it is not at all uncommon to suffer from multiple allergies—to one or more foods, to pollen, to housedust, to animal danders, to insect venom. The person who finds himself in such a fix has a hard time trying to avoid all the things that make him ill.

Other factors affect allergy in general, although normally not allergy to insects. Oddly enough, sudden changes of temperature and weather, such as a cold front moving through an area, may trigger allergy symptoms. It is the abruptness of the change rather than the temperature or kind of weather that appears to act as the trigger. Even the state of one's emotions can affect one's sensitivity to allergens. Emotional stress such as anger or anxiety can cause actual physical changes within the body that lower its tolerance to allergenic substances.

The concept of tolerance to allergens in the environment, together with the idea that the above factors constitute cumulative "allergic load," seems to explain best why some of us react with allergy diseases to essentially harmless substances while others of us do not and why allergic individuals sometimes react with relatively mild symptoms or none at all and at other times react with severe symptoms. Again, while this concept does not necessarily always apply to allergy to insects, it helps explain the general nature of allergy. Let us take a quick look at it.

It has been said that anyone can be made allergic to something if the conditions (the allergic load) are such as to overcome his tolerance. The allergic person simply has a lower tolerance level than the nonallergic person. He becomes more easily sensitized to allergenic substances in his environment, and thus he usually reacts more readily when factors such as we just discussed are present. We can illustrate the concept of tolerance and the allergic load with the following drawing. The "tolerance truck" pictured here was built to carry just so much—in this case, a quarter of a ton, or 500 pounds:

Allergic Load   *Tolerance Level*

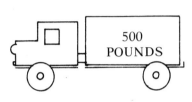

250 pounds allergens (pollen, mold, housedust, insect debris, etc.)

100 pounds worth of sudden weather change, such as cold front moving through

100 pounds worth of emotional stress such as anxiety before an exam or job interview

 50 pounds worth of slight infection (common cold or the like)

500 pounds

Allergic Load   *Tolerance Level Breached*

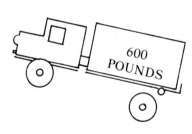

BREAKDOWN!
(allergy symptoms appear)

350 pounds allergens (pollen, mold, housedust, insect debris, plus insect venom from two stings)

100 pounds worth of sudden weather change

100 pounds worth of emotional stress

 50 pounds worth of slight infection

600 pounds

How do we differentiate an allergic reaction to an insect sting or bite from a normal reaction? A normal reaction involves only the immediate area of the bite or sting. Usually it consists of a wheal, some pain, and quite a bit of itching. There may be some swelling contiguous to the wound itself. An allergic reaction produces symptoms in areas removed from the site of the sting or bite and may involve one or more body systems, such as the respiratory, gastrointestinal, cardiac, and skin. Thus the allergic individual may not only have pain, a wheal, itching at the sting or bite site but also feel nauseated, weak, and sweaty. He may suffer breathing difficulties. He may break out in widespread hives. His blood pressure may fall. His heartbeat may increase. He may go into shock.

Can the doctor know ahead of time who may suffer a severe allergic reaction? So far, unless a person has already been sensitized by a sting or a bite in the past, there is no test to determine who will be allergic to insects. Once sensitized, however, the allergic individual presents his physician with some clues. Skin tests play an important role in the diagnosis of many allergies. Such tests are relatively simple procedures. A bit of an extract made from the allergenic substance under suspicion is either rubbed unto a tiny scratch made on the patient's skin or injected just beneath the skin. If the individual is allergic a red wheal like a hive or mosquito bite will appear at the site. Usually the more allergic the patient is, the more positive the reaction. Skin tests are not quite as reliable in diagnosing allergy to insects as in diagnosing allergy to some other allergens, such as pollens and mold. But in conjunction with the patient's medical history and his account of earlier stings or bites and the subsequent symptoms, skin tests provide the physician with necessary clues. I will discuss the problems of diagnosis of reactions to specific insects as I discuss the insects themselves in later chapters.

There are also certain characteristics that persons allergic to insects seem to share. In a study of patients allergic to insects who suffered generalized systemic reactions about half of them also suffered from hay fever, asthma, or other allergies, and there was a history of allergy in their families. Of those under age twenty the majority were males. After age twenty the proportions of female subjects rose.

To end this chapter on a cheerful note, let me hasten to point out that the endangered are relatively few in number and that for most of us insects are little more than seasonal pests. We are ordinarily willing to let the doctors and the health authorities worry about insects' role as disease vectors and the farmers and the Department of Agriculture worry about their role as crop despoilers. Even so, since few of us will get through life unscathed, we should know a bit about the insects that attack us, how to treat the wounds they inflict, and how to avoid their attack if we can. "Know the enemy" was always a wise slogan.

READER'S GUIDE TO INSECT ALLERGY

1. Allergy is an abnormal reaction to substances ordinarily harmless to most people.

2. Factors that contribute to the production of allergy symptoms—though not necessarily to allergy to insects—are:

   • Duration and amount of exposure to allergenic substances
   • Nature of allergenic substance
   • Presence of underlying disease or infection
   • Temperature and weather changes
   • Emotional stress

3. The production of allergy symptoms depends in great part upon the individual's "allergic load" and tolerance level.

4. Most people do not exhibit other than normal reactions to insect stings or bites. Only a few suffer severe allergic, or generalized systemic, reactions. Yet such reactions can be fatal.

5. An individual can suffer from more than one allergy. A person can have hay fever, for instance, and also suffer from allergy headaches. About one-third of my patients who are allergic to insect stings are also allergic to penicillin injections.

3
" . . . And the Bees"

Bees, the instruments of Mr. J's unhappy initiation into the drawbacks of country living, belong to the highly developed order Hymenoptera. They and their cousins—wasps, hornets, yellow jackets, and ants—can be numbered among man's best friends, and they are among his worst enemies as far as insect allergy is concerned. In general, throughout most of our country the bright world of summer sun, of spring showers, and of Indian summer buzzes with the Hymenoptera's frenzied activity. From about the middle of April until the middle of October—December down in my country in the mountains of western North Carolina—they are everywhere, building nests, gathering food, and propagating their kind. In all this strenous industry they are very likely to cross paths with human beings.

Of the estimated 100,000 different species in the order of Hymenoptera, we will be most concerned with the honeybee, the yellow jacket, the Polistes wasp, the hornet, the fire ant, and the red harvester ant, for these are the most common culprits in man's collisions with the stinger insects.

Hymenoptera are stingers. There is a not-too-subtle difference between stinging insects and biting insects. The stingers usually inject venom into their victim much as a doctor or nurse might inject with a hypodermic needle, and they produce severe reactions more frequently than do the biters. With a few exceptions the biters do their damage with the saliva that they dispense through their mouthparts. As seems natural, the biters approach their victim head first, whereas the stingers usually inject from their hind ends. The victim, however, rarely knows which end hit him. Often enough he does not even know what bit or stung him. That can cause a good deal of difficulty in diagnosis and treatment.

The stinging apparatus possessed by the females of the Hymenoptera clan is the cause of all the havoc and pain. The mechanism is similar in all the species of the order. It consists of a sort of double-barreled syringe, a hollow needlelike stinger with two lancets. The stinging insect thrusts the lancets into the victim's flesh. They not only penetrate but also pump venom from the poison sac down the hollow canal of the stinger. The honeybee's lancets differ from those of her cousins in that they are barbed. She can sting another insect and withdraw to go her own way again, but when she encounters tough human hide, the barbs will not let go. In her struggles to free herself, or when the victim angrily brushes her away, the stinging apparatus, venom sac and all, is torn from her abdomen. Gutted, she will die. Meanwhile, the reflexive action of the lancets continues to drive the venom deeper into the victim's wound. No matter what, the bee gets in the last blow. Oddly, the queen bee's lancets are not barbed; thus she can sting more than once. Wasps and yellow jackets are equally fortunate. Having no barbs upon their lancets, they too can fly away to sting another day.

It is estimated that there are about five thousand different species of bees in North America, some of which range all the way to the northern borders of Greenland. Contrary to what we learned as schoolchildren about the fascinating society of honeybees, most bees are solitary. They live alone and like it. Their pattern of life, while it varies from species to species, follows a common line. They build their nests in the ground, store provisions in the nest for the egg or eggs that they lay, then seal the nest and vanish, leaving the eggs on their own. When the larvae hatch, they eat the food stores, become pupae, and then emerge from the nests as adults to go their own separate ways and repeat the process. Among the more familiar solitary bees are the large carpenter bees, which can bore holes in wood a half inch in diameter, and the leaf-cutting bees, so called because they cut leaves to line their nests. The latter can do some damage to plants, but have proved helpful to man. In Saskatchewan, Canada, not too long ago farmers discovered that, when they cut down the wild forests bordering their fields, their alfalfa acres away from the tree stands went unpollinated. The leaf cutters needed the trees for their habitat and pollinated only in their immediate area. How often we learn the hard way.

The most familiar and fascinating bee is, of course, the honeybee. Few of us reach the end of our school days without learning of its astonishing social development, including its method of communicating with its fellows. We learn that the honeybee executes an elaborate dance on the threshold of the hive to tell her companions where and how far the nearest food supply is. We learn that the hive itself is a tight ship in which every bee knows its place and its job. We also learn that without bees man would be literally fruitless. Honeybees are first-class pollinators. Without their prodigious efforts our orchards would be sterile, as would be many of our flowers, crops, and clovers. And, of course, we would not have honey.

We know that the queen bee is the key to the colony's future and that drone bees lead an easy, privileged life up until their brief mating flight into the wild blue yonder, which ends with the fertilizing of the queen and the death of the drones. The survival of the colony depends on the relentless labors of the worker bees, who are all sterile females. The more we learn about the bee, the more we respect it. It is astonishing that a creature which is so small that many of us are mistakenly inclined to consider it brainless can be so highly organized and so successful.

The organization of the hive is truly startling. As many as eighty or ninety thousand bees may inhibit one colony, a number guaranteed to ensure chaos if bees did not follow inherent laws of cooperation and order. A worker bee, for instance, emerges from its cell as an adult to begin life as a janitor. She has no other choice. She moves automatically to the cleanup squad, with whom for about ten days she cleans out empty cells, removes dead companions, and in general keeps house furiously. Then, for the next ten days or so, she moves into a new job as nursemaid. During this period she converts pollen from the hive's storehouse into royal jelly, which she deposits on the hive floor for the larvae to consume. Queen bees receive this food, which is apparently a treat, all their lives, but plebian larvae get it for only three days. They must then turn to honey and pollen for their sustenance. Interestingly, drone larvae, which develop from unfertilized eggs, get only honey following their allotment of royal jelly. Perhaps this sweet diet is compensation for the shortness of their pleasant lives.

The lucky, or unlucky, drone (depending upon your view of such things) who is successful on his mating flight dies in the act of copulation; his genitals are torn out by the queen as she leaves him. The drones that never accomplish their purpose in life almost always die soon also. Unable to care for themselves, they starve because the worker bees kick them out of the hive when food stores are depleted. Unhappily too for the drones, beekeepers have devised a way to inseminate the queen artificially, making drones even more of a surplus than nature intended. The introduction of an artificially inseminated queen into a hive is interesting. She can be introduced only into a queenless hive, for a resident queen would soon kill her. But even the workers of a queenless hive may not accept a new queen, may even throw her out, if they do not have time to be introduced properly. So the beekeeper places her in a small, screened box, the entrance of which is corked with candy. By the time the workers have eaten their way through the treat, the inseminated queen has had time to absorb the hive's characteristic odor, which automatically makes her one of them.

But back to the worker bee. After her stint as nursemaid she begins to take short flights from the hive, which are somewhat educational in nature. She is becoming acquainted with the terrain, so to speak. She moves out into the new field of endeavor because her wax-making glands have matured at the expense of her royal-jelly-making glands, and she is no longer physically capable of functioning as a nursemaid, although she can regenerate the proper equipment if the need arises and once again tend to the larvae, which are the key to the colony's survival. In between the educational flights in which she tries out her wings, the worker may act as a builder, constructing new combs, or she may act as a security guard against the invasions of other insects, bears, or human beings.

At the end of this stage the worker moves out into the ranks of the busy bees who comb the countryside for nectar and pollen, who, in the process, cross-pollinate our flowers, our fruits, and a number of our important crops. (As every gardener knows, if you do not have bees, you will have no cucumbers, no matter how healthy your vines.) Unfortunately, human beings are often shortsighted. Bee populations all over the world are on the decline because of the use of herbicides and insecticides and because we have plowed up our fields of wild flowers or paved them over with concrete. The nectar of wild flowers is the bees' main sustenance. Knowing this, the wise gardener will either let a stand of wild flowers grow near his neatly turned plot or will plant nectar-rich flowers to attract his bee friends. The dearth of bees among Florida orange groves, for instance, has become so serious in recent years that a small business of transporting hives to the area has sprung up. Not long ago in Utah beekeepers instituted a suit against the federal government when the Air Force killed off their bees by spraying insecticide in the area.

Because bees are becoming scarce, beekeeping and renting out beehives to farmers have become very profitable, so profitable that in remote areas (especially in California) bee rustlers have moved in to cart away beehives and colonies in toto from their stands. Some beekeepers have put brands on their hives or wired them for burglar alarms.

"...And the Bees"

Bees are important! By the time the worker moves out into the world, she is capable of flying as far as eight miles from the hive to return with a load equal to half her own body weight. She can do all this at a speed of twenty-five miles an hour, but being smarter than we might think, she is likely to fly home at lesser speeds with a few rest stops on the way. It has been estimated, although I cannot imagine how, that the worker bees of a single hive will travel the equivalent of a dozen times around the world to produce one pound of honey. Their hard-working lives are short; they are lucky if they survive more than six weeks.

The queen bee deserves the special attention she gets, it would seem, for she is capable of laying 1,800 eggs a day at the height of the bee season. The bulk of the eggs is greater than her own weight. She lays one egg in each of the wax cells the workers have built. In fact, they carefully lead her around as she goes about her work, laying worker eggs in the smaller cells, drone eggs in the larger. She will live three or four years in the colony doing nothing but laying eggs. The number of eggs is controlled by the amount of food the workers give her, which may be a form of bee birth control. When her egg-laying capacity is exhausted, she will suffer the fate nature has in store for the surplus and the used-up: either she will be thrown out of the hive by the workers to starve or a new, young queen bee will dispatch her with a sting. Done in by her own daughter!

Male chauvinists may wonder that tens of thousands of females of any kind can live and work so closely and in such harmony to ensure the survival of their species. Feminists may retort that it is only possible because the males disappear so early from the scene. Whatever, there is surely a lesson in the honeybees' cooperation and the ability of the species to work together. For example, when the temperature goes down and the honeybees grow cold, they cluster in a ball. The bees on the outside are gradually worked toward the center of the ball and the warmth, while the warm center bees move to the outside to take their turn being chilly. One for all and all for one.

Insects and Allergy

While honeybees will attack savagely if their hive is disturbed, ordinarily they do not bother human beings if unprovoked. Beekeepers report that some bees in a hive are more irritable and aggressive than others and more inclined to sting. Bees out gathering nectar after a rain are more likely to be irritable and to sting anything that gets in their way, because the rain has washed away a good part of their food supply. Certain odors, for instance, those of leather and suede, seem to irritate them also. Frustrated bees should be avoided; busy bees should be left undisturbed.

Bees have their problems with their fellow insects too. They can be seized by robber flies in mid-flight, sucked dry of their vital fluids, and dropped as dry husks to the ground. Certain spiders and certain bugs, aptly named ambush bugs, lie in wait within flowers to dine on the bees. One kind of fly waits near the hive to catch a passing bee, and lay an egg between the segments of its abdomen. Although the bee is then freed to go its way, it bears a slow death with it, for the egg soon hatches into a maggot that dines within. Other parasites and diseases attack the larvae in their cells. The honeybee has a good many enemies other than the human race.

Having now treated the interesting life of the honeybee with a bit of sympathy, and having remarked upon their beneficial, vital roles in our continued welfare, I must now turn to the darker side of the picture, the hazard they can present. Unfortunately, from the killer bee down to the lowliest domesticated honeybee, bees can kill.

READER'S GUIDE TO THE HONEYBEE
AND BUMBLEBEE

The honeybee and the bumble bee are the two common species of bee that most of us will encounter in the United States:

- The honeybee's body is so thickly covered with fine hairs that it appears fuzzy. Its color ranges from light brown to black. (See Plates 1 and 2.)
- The bumblebee is large and heavy-bodied with thick hair over its body. Yellow and black in coloring, it makes a buzzing noise in flights. (See Plate 3.)

HONEYBEES AND BUMBLEBEES

4

The Hazard
of Bees

The killer bee represents the ultimate hazard in the Hymenoptera clan. We have heard a lot about this aggressive bee which is coming to us out of Africa by way of Brazil. Articles have been written about its savage nature, newspapers have headlined its approach to the United States, a frightening TV documentary showed it in action. Unfortunately, the potential reality rates every scary picture and headline: they are killers, and they are coming our way at an estimated rate of two hundred miles a year. They are supposed to arrive in the United States in the 1980s unless something happens to stop them—a disease, for instance, or the sudden rise of a natural predator. It is just possible that their bellicose nature may be watered down over time by mingling with the less-aggressive native honeybees.

Why were they ever let out of Africa? The idea was to bring them to Brazil to cross with the ordinary honeybee (which came to us originally from Europe) in order to obtain a greater production of honey. The vicious African bee produces about 50 percent more honey than the European honeybee. Thus man, ever on the lookout for the bigger and better, tampered with nature, thinking to turn a better profit. Unhappily for the Brazilian people, some of the African bee swarms, complete with their queens, escaped and spread out over the countryside. In 1980, a generation later, it is estimated that there will be thousands of these colonies wild in Brazil. They have crossed with the Brazilian bees, but as is so often the way, the bad trait is dominant, and the hybrids are as savage as their African ancestors. The colonies are moving north. On their way they have killed a good many chickens, dogs, and larger livestock, and several people.

In one town killer bees attacked children in a park and had to be driven off with flamethrowers. In a mass attack at Sao Paulo, Brazil, swarms so large that they turned the day dark stung over five hundred people and killed a large number of chickens. They attacked an army barracks and sent the sentries on the run. The threat of the killer bees is not that their venom is more toxic than that of ordinary honeybees, it is that they attack en masse, injecting near-lethal and lethal doses of venom. As we noted in Chapter 1, the toxic effects of 500 to 800 beestings can kill. Scientists from the National Academy of Sciences of the United States traveled to Brazil to look into the problem. They found that killer bees stung a small leather ball that bounced about near their hive ninety-two times within five seconds. Such rapidity does not allow much time to escape. The killer bees also have a reputation for flying faster and pursuing their victims farther than ordinary bees. 2107002

Well, let us wait to worry about the killer bees until they get here. Some of us have worries enough right here at home with our own garden variety of honeybee. Countless millions of bees are flying around, going about their business. Relatively few cross paths with human beings. When they do, the endangered person is the exception rather than the rule. Even so, an estimated four out of every thousand people could suffer a severe, even fatal, allergic reaction to a honeybee sting or the sting of another species of Hymenoptera. This opens up an awful lot of grim possibilities. As I stated earlier, more people die annually from the effects of insect stings and bites than from snakebites. The victims of insect allergy number only in the dozens each year, but since most of those fatalities depend more on the victim's sensitivity to insect venom or substances in insect saliva than on the toxicity of multiple stings, such deaths can and should be prevented. Deaths from snakebite occur almost exclusively because of the toxic effects of the venom, although the severity of the victim's reaction may depend in part upon his health and age and the location of the bite. It is also likely that there are more fatalities annually due to allergy to insects than are officially recorded because the victims often are listed as having "died of natural causes" or of "death due to heart failure."

Admittedly, most people suffer only momentary discomfort when stung by a bee. Such a reaction is the norm. A pinprick of pain—much the same sort of pain one feels when an inexperienced nurse wields a hypodermic needle—is followed by the appearance of a small red wheal or hive at the sting site, surrounded by a whitish area. Perhaps a little heat develops in the area, and usually a somewhat fierce itch. All is soon forgotten even if the bee itself is not forgiven.

The reaction of some individuals, however, is a bit more than normal. The area around the sting site may swell and remain swollen for a few hours or even a day before subsiding. This sort of reaction is called a *local reaction* to differentiate it from the normal. As long as the swelling departs reasonably soon, there is little cause for anxiety. But if the swebling intensifies, feels hot, and does not depart, a physician should be consulted. There is always the chance of secondary infection with an insect sting or bite. Even if infection is not present, if the swelling is considerable—for example, if it covers two joints of an arm or leg—I recommend that the victim see his doctor so that the possibility of his being allergic can be assessed.

The location of the sting can present special problems. Stings in the throat, the mouth, and the nose area can cause more than normal distress, especially if swelling is pronounced. Stings close to the eye are especially dangerous, since a pronounced local reaction can injure the eye. Stings on the eyelid may penetrate to injure the eyeball, or the stinger, if not removed, may work its way through the lid to affect the eye. It is wise to see a physician if one is stung in the

(*Text continues on page 51.*)

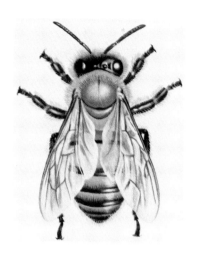

Plate 1.
Honeybees (×4).
The honeybee's
body is so thickly
covered with fine
hairs that it appears
fuzzy. Its color
ranges from light
brown to black.
*Courtesy of Merck
Sharp & Dohme, Di-
vision of Merck &
Co., Inc.*

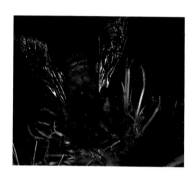

Plate 2.
Honeybee foraging
on burdock.
*Courtesy of E. M.
Barrows.*

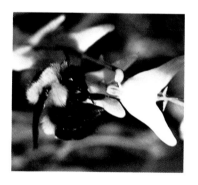

Plate 3.
Bumblebee.
The bumblebee is
large and heavy-
bodied with thick
hair over the body.
Yellow and black in
coloring, it makes a
buzzing noise in
flight.
*Courtesy of E. M.
Barrows.*

35

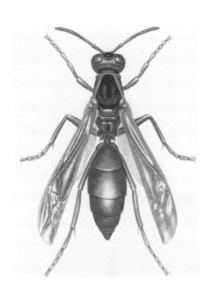

Plate 4.
Wasp (×2). Usually reddish brown in color, the Polistes is slender with a spindle-shaped abdomen. Its nest consists of a single tier of cells, is more or less circular in appearance, and is attached by a thin stalk, often under barn and house eaves.
Courtesy of Merck Sharpe & Dohme, Division of Merck & Co., Inc.

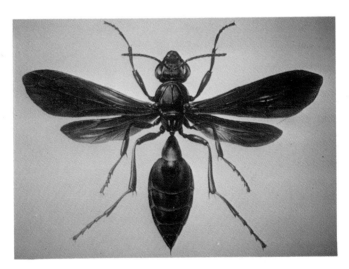

Plate 5.
Paper wasp.
Courtesy of Center for Disease Control.

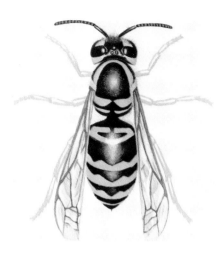

Plate 6.
Yellow jacket (×4).
Smaller than the wasp,
the yellow jacket has
black and yellow stripes
much like those of the
hornet. Its nest consists of
several tiers of cells and
is often to be found in old
posts, stumps, and holes
in the ground.
*Courtesy of Merck Sharpe
& Dohme, Division of
Merck & Co., Inc.*

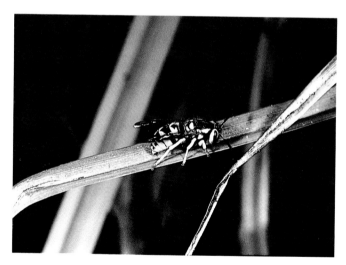

Plate 7.
Yellow jacket.
Courtesy of Dr. C. L. Hogue.

37

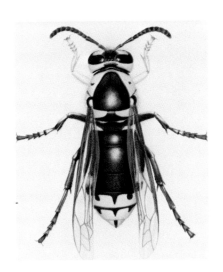

Plate 8.
Hornet (×3). The most familiar species is large and black with yellowish-white markings. The nests are large and football-shaped and commonly hang from the branches of a tree or bush, although sometimes they are built in grass.
Courtesy of Merck Sharpe & Dohme, Division of Merck & Co., Inc.

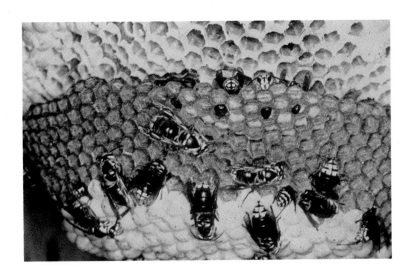

Plate 9.
Bald-faced hornets on nest.
Courtesy of Center for Disease Control.

38

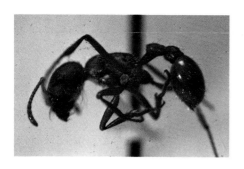

Plate 10.
Harvester ant. Black
or red in color, the
harvester is long-
legged and often as
large as ⅓ inch.
*Courtesy of Center
Laboratories, Inc.*

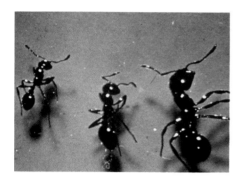

Plate 11.
Imported fire ant.
Fire ants are 4 to 6
millimeters in size
and usually red in
color. They appear
to take on the
coloration of the soil
of their habitat:
dark soil, dark ants;
black soil, black
ants. The nests are
mounds of various
heights depending
upon the
surroundings.
*Courtesy of Center
for Disease Control
and John Ridley and
courtesy of W. L.
Watson, M.D.*

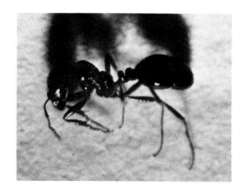

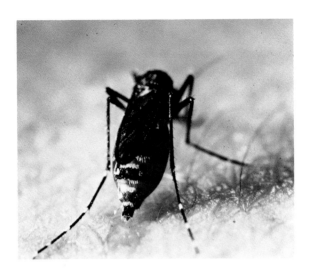

Plate 12.
Mosquito. Mosquitoes come in various sizes
and colors, but all have round heads, a slender
proboscis, antennae, and palpi, or feelers.
*Courtesy of United States Department of
Agriculture.*

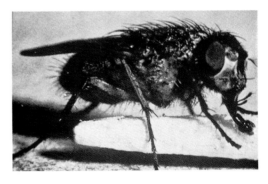

Plate 13.
Housefly. The housefly is short of body,
bristly, and somewhat plump with see-
through wings.
Courtesy of A. H. Robins Co.

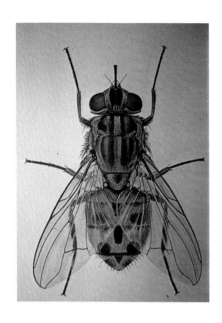

Plate 14.
Stable fly. The stable fly
is about the same size
and color as the housefly,
but a little larger in the
body.
*Courtesy of Darryl
Sanders.*

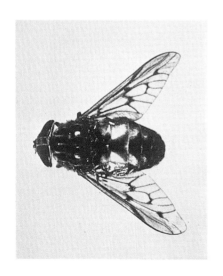

Plate 15.
Horsefly. The horsefly is
large and heavy-bodied,
ranging in size from 16 to
28 millimeters. Some are
all black, and some are
black and white. The
latter are more of a pest
for livestock than for
human beings.
*Courtesy of Center for
Disease Control.*

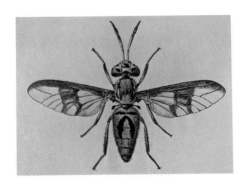

Plate 16.
Deerfly. Deerflies are smaller than horseflies—8 to 10 millimeters in length. Some are black with yellowish spots on the sides of their abdomens, and some are gray or yellowish-gray with black spots along their abdomens. The former are almost everywhere, the latter are more common in the western United States.
Courtesy of Center for Disease Control.

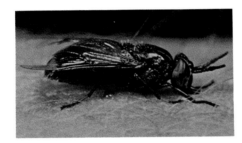

Plate 17.
Black deerfly.
Courtesy of Clemson University Extension Service, United States Department of Agriculture.

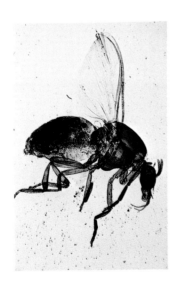

Plate 18.
Blackfly. Small—between 1 and 5 millimeters in length—with coloring that ranges from black to gray, the blackfly has short, broad wings and thick legs. Its most distinctive feature is a humpbacked appearance.
Courtesy of Harry Most, M.D.

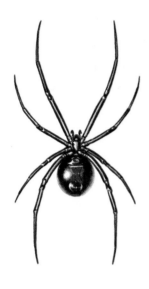

Plate 19.
Female black-widow spider
(×1½). The female black
widow is black and has a
shiny, fat, roundish abdomen
with a red or orange hourglass
marking on the underside.
*Courtesy of Merck Sharpe &
Dohme, Division of Merck &
Co., Inc., and United States
Department of Agriculture.*

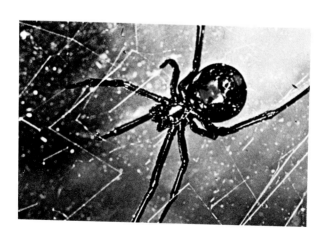

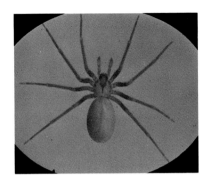

Plate 20.
Brown-recluse spider
(×2). The female brown
recluse ranges in color
from dark brown to tan. A
characteristic darker
fiddle-shaped mark runs
back from the area of her
eyes almost to her
abdomen.
*Courtesy of Hugh L.
Keegan.*

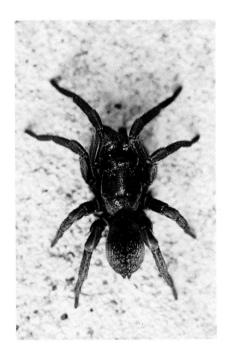

Plate 21.
Tarantula. The tarantula
is large, hairy, and black
or brown in color with
legs several inches long.
*Courtesy of Hugh L.
Keegan.*

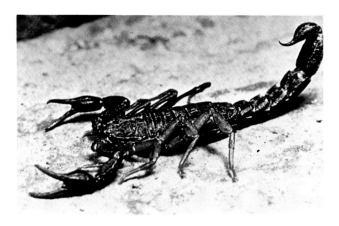

Plate 22.
Scorpion. The scorpion looks like a very small lobster or crayfish. It is gray, black, or yellowish in color and varies in length from ½ inch to 8 inches. The poisonous species have lemon-yellow or greenish-yellow coloring in the tail area, where the stinger is located.
Courtesy of United States Department of Agriculture.

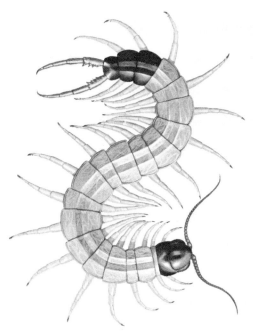

Plate 23.
Centipede (slightly smaller than actual size). *Courtesy of Merck Sharp & Dohme, Division of Merck & Co., Inc.*

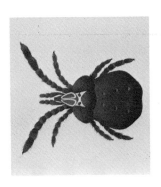

Plate 24.
Chigger larva (×90). The larva may be seen by the naked eye as a tiny red spot or pinpoint in or around the center of the reddened area of the bite. *Courtesy of Merck Sharpe & Dohme, Division of Merck & Co., Inc.*

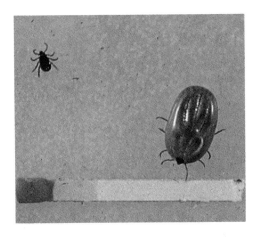

Plate 25.
Dog ticks before and after engorging. The most common tick species is flat and hard-bodied with six legs in the larva stage and eight in the adult. When engorged, the female is grayish in color and can be as large as ½ inch. There are also soft-bodied species that feed rapidly on human beings much as bedbugs do. *Courtesy of National Pest Control Association.*

46

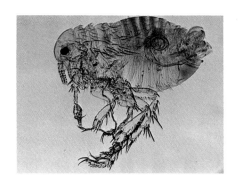

Plate 26.
Male flea (×15). Fleas are brown, wingless, and hard-bodied with long, slender legs. *Courtesy of Hugh L. Keegan.*

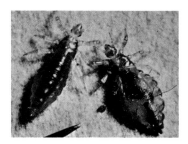

Plate 27.
Male and female body lice (×15). Lice are tiny in size and gray or dirty white in color. *Courtesy of Center for Disease Control.*

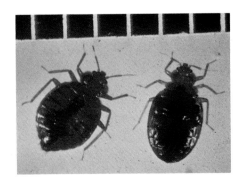

Plate 28.
Bedbugs. Bedbugs
are flat and reddish
brown in color,
changing to red
when engorged with
blood. They are 4 to
5 millimeters in
length and 3 mil-
limeters in breadth.
*Courtesy of Center
for Disease Control.*

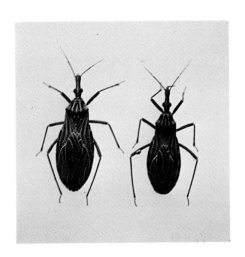

Plate 29.
Kissing bugs. The
kissing bug is flat
and brown or black
in color with an
average length
between 18 and 24
millimeters. Some
species flaunt
orange markings.
*Courtesy of Hugh L.
Keegan.*

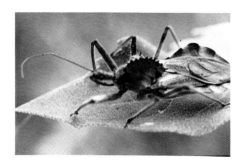

Plate 30.
Wheel bug. The wheel bug is mouse gray in color and may be as large as 1 to 1¼ inches. It has a distinctive crest over the head that looks like part of a cog or a geared wheel.
Courtesy of E. M. Barrows.

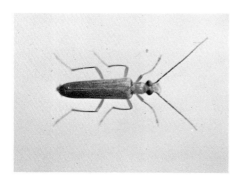

Plate 31.
Blister beetle. The blister beetle ranges in size from ¼ inch to 1 inch. It is somewhat soft of body and has a rather broad head and narrow neck. Blister beetles in the eastern United States are purplish in color. Those in the West are commonly ash gray.
Courtesy of Hugh L. Keegan.

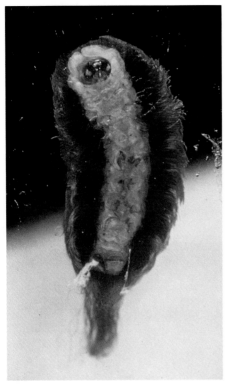

Plate 32.
Puss caterpillar
(*Above*, top view;
below, bottom view).
The puss caterpillar
is shaped like a
teardrop because of
its pointed tail. It is
tan, darkish gray,
and cream in color
and anywhere from
½ to 1½ inches in
length.
*Courtesy of Center
for Disease Control.*

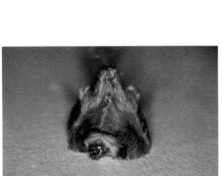

The Hazard of Bees

above areas, just to play it safe and to prevent possible permanent and serious consequences.

The greatest hazards of bee venom are presented by multiple stings and the danger of an allergic, or generalized systemic, reaction. Let us consider another example of the toxicity of multiple stings besides that of the gentleman in Chapter 1 who strolled along an African riverbank and was attacked by thousands of bees. A case was reported by a physician some time ago of a young army officer who landed among a swarm of bees when he jumped onto a ledge. He tried to escape along the ledge as "thousands" of bees stung him on every exposed part of his body. Exhausted by fear and pain, he fell from the ledge with the bees following him down. They even crawled into his nose, ears, and mouth to sting. He lost consciousness, and when he revived, he was horribly ill and too weak to move. The bees continued to swarm over him, but apparently ceased stinging. He was discovered shortly after the attack and rushed to a hospital. Swelling of his head, tongue, ears, neck, hands, and wrists was exceedingly pronounced, and his flesh was dark with embedded stingers. Many of the wounds were already pus-laden and oozing. Over 300 stingers were removed from his eyelids, tongue, and lips, and about 300 more from his scalp. Meanwhile the swelling increased until his lips, nose, eyelids, and ears were almost three times their normal size. I am happy to record that, after this gruesome ordeal, treatment was successful and the young officer's life was saved. All in all, however, he was made very sick and had a very close call.

The severely allergic can have just as close a call from the sting of one bee. For example, a colleague of mine sent me the following case:

> Ronnie, age eight, was riding his bicycle home in the evening. . . . He came to a sprinkler, opened his mouth to take in a drink of water, and got an angry honeybee instead. It stung him on the inner surface of the upper lip. He was hurt and scared and raced for home.
> On the way he developed generalized urticaria [hives]. By the time he arrived, he was gasping for breath. His father, fortunately, was quick to understand—and act. He took his knife and released

51

the stinger and ran for my office with Ronnie. Ronnie had severe angioneurotic edema [swelling] by his arrival. He also had no blood pressure and was a little cyanotic [bluish or grayish from a deficiency of oxygen in the blood].

I had my nurse call for an ambulance, while I gave Ronnie the first of several "hypos" of epinephrine, plus oxygen and intravenous Decadron. He spent the night in the hospital under observation. . . . Next day he was OK and was discharged. . . . I am told that he had a severe local reaction to a beesting several years ago.[1]

Thus the allergic are endangered. For them the insect world presents a special threat. The bee that pollinates their flower gardens and apple trees may send them to the hospital, or worse.

What are the symptoms of an *allergic, or generalized systemic, reaction?* The symptoms may begin mildly enough with a dry cough, itching and swelling about the eyes, sneezing, wheezing, and widespread hives. Even if matters go no further than this, one who has suffered such symptoms following a beesting, or the sting or bite of any other insect, should consult a physician, for, as we shall see later in this chapter, there are protective measures that should be taken against the chance of a far more severe reaction following a future sting.

If the symptoms progress beyond the mild stage, the victim's pulse may become rapid, and his skin either very pale or flushed, and his blood pressure may fall. He may feel a constriction in his throat and chest, and his breathing may become difficult. His symptoms will rapidly worsen, and he will feel increasing unease and a sense of impending disaster, even of death. All this may be accompanied by other manifestations, such as abdominal cramps, diarrhea, nausea, vomiting, chills and fever, collapse, loss of consciousness, and a bloody, frothy sputum. As we noted earlier, a severe allergic reaction can take the victim from sting to fatal anaphylactic shock within ten or fifteen minutes or even sooner. Thus even the first mild symptoms should be treated as an emergency,

[1]Charles E. Connor, M.D., Cashmere, Washington.

The Hazard of Bees

and the victim should be gotten to medical aid as quickly as possible. There is no time to lose.

There is also such a thing as a *delayed, serum-sickness reaction*. Such a reaction usually occurs ten to fourteen days after a sting, and its symptoms can range from mild to severe. They can include headache, general malaise, fever, lymph-gland involvement, and painful joints that resemble arthritis. There are a few unfortunate individuals who suffer not only an immediate reaction but also a delayed one later, a form of double jeopardy. A delayed reaction may be puzzling to patient and physician alike if the patient has forgotten the initial sting. It is not certain whether immediate and delayed reactions are part and parcel of the same general mechanism or two separate entities. We do know that the delayed reaction is less severe.

There is one more type of reaction, one that I hope no reader of this book will suffer simply from his, or her, exposure to the information accumulated here. We are creatures open to suggestion, some of us more than others. Thus there is such a thing as a *psychological reaction* to an insect sting or bite, which is sparked by pure fright. Perhaps the victim saw a headline, "Man Dies After Single Beesting!", or perhaps a relative landed in a hospital emergency room after being stung. In any case, the imagination goes to work upon the body to develop an array of symptoms, such as rapid heartbeat, quick and shallow breathing, a feeling of weakness, dizziness, and the like. It is even possible for such a reaction to be fatal, for the victim may simply die of fright.

If I, like a Paul Revere of medicine, have alerted the reader to the dangers inherent in allergy to beestings (or the stings or bites of other insects), the reader will probably ask: How do you identify the allergic? How do you pick out that four in a thousand who could become grim statistics?

Unfortunately, this has not been easy for the physician, or even the allergy specialist, to do. As mentioned earlier, we have no single reliable test to pinpoint allergy to insect venom. Skin testing, which is employed effectively in diagnosing allergies to substances such as pollen and mold, is helpful, but it often fails to distinguish those who are allergic to insect stings and bites. Thus it cannot be totally relied upon. Assuming curiosity on the part of my reader, I will disgress a bit here to explain how skin tests are conducted.

Two types of skin tests are usually employed to determine the extent of a patient's allergy to insects: the scratch, or prick, test and the intradermal test. These tests are especially helpful to the allergist in deciding upon an injection schedule to desensitize, or immunize, the patient against further stings. In the *scratch test* a small scratch is made on the skin, to which is applied a tiny amount of a dilute extract that is usually made from ground-up whole insect bodies. Frequently in testing for Hymenoptera allergy, allergists use a mixture of wasp, honeybee, yellow jacket, and hornet. Or they may use an extract made from one or another of those species alone. If the patient is allergic to bees (or the other stingers), a hive or wheal or rash will appear at the site. If the scratch test proves negative, the allergist will probably try an *intradermal skin test*, which is a bit more potent and could produce a systemic reaction in the severely allergic individual. In the intradermal test a small amount of the extract is injected into the upper layer of skin with a hypodermic needle. As with the scratch test a wheal or hive or rash indicates a positive, allergic reaction.

Recent research has focused on the extracts used in testing in order to make the procedure a more reliable measure of an individual's sensitivity to bee venom. One of the difficulties with the whole-body extract used in diagnostic skin testing is that the extracts are not standardized. Some contain more of the insect's venom and venom sac than do others. As a result researchers have initiated a method of testing that uses venom alone in extracts. The method is not yet universally employed because extracting venom is a more difficult process than grinding up whole bodies. In some cases the bees— or other stinging insects—are electrically stimulated to sting, and the venom collected. In others the sacs are removed, and the venom drawn out by capillary action.

Very recently another testing technique, which may someday supplant skin testing, has been introduced. It is called RAST, short for *Radioallergosorbent Test*, which is a mouthful. It measures the IgE antibodies in a patient's serum.

Since none of the diagnostic tests is totally reliable, the allergist must combine the results with the patient's own history: his description or identification of what stung him and the symptoms that resulted; his account of previous stings and the sort of symptoms that they produced; and the diagnosis of other allergies. Two things make it difficult for the allergist to pin down the details of the patient's account. Many people do not know one insect from another and will label everything that stings a bee. And many people will play down their symptoms, not realizing the importance attached to even mild symptoms of a systemic reaction. They are not aware that another time such symptoms are likely to be anything but mild.

The bee frequently leaves its trademark behind in the form of a stinger and venom sac. Thus its sting is the easiest to identify. It has given its all, so to speak, and either the patient or the doctor will be able to scrape the evidence from the wound. The other stinging insects usually take their stingers with them as they make their escape. Ideally, of course, the alert victim brings in the body of the enemy, either squashed or intact, so that positive identification can be made. Also, if the victim has been messing around beehives or if he has bumped into a football-sized papier-maché object hanging from a tree or if he has been knocking wasps' nests out from under the eaves of his home, the allergist has a pretty solid clue.

I keep a set of slides of the common stinging and biting insects to help prod my patients' memories. I even have some handsome insects trapped in amber. Often, however, to no avail because one insect looks like every other insect to the patient, who typically says, "I guess it was just a bee, Dr. Frazier. It sure looked like a bee." One thing is certain: it hurt like a bee.

The recording of symptoms of earlier stings and bites is a harder nut to crack. Human beings simply do not like to admit that they can be bested by a bug. "Sure, it stung a little," they say bravely. "Yep, it got pretty swollen. Well, yes, I did feel sort of funny." Weaklike, you know, and it was hard to get my breath." And so on. For example, I have a tennis-playing friend who represents the epitome of machismo: virile, inordinately healthy, he is of the chest-beating stripe, swearing often and loudly that he has never been ill a day in his life (particularly in the presence of doctors, who, I am sure, he considers supernumeraries). Nevertheless, he was taken to the emergency room of a local hospital not so long ago after he had been stung by two bees while out trimming a hedge. When he recovered from anaphylactic shock, saved only by heroic efforts on the part of the emergency-room personnel, he confided that he had been meaning to come to see me. He said:

> I know you're an allergist, Claude, and I know you fellows exaggerate every little thing, but I was going to ask you about something that happened to me earlier in the summer when I took the family camping in the Great Smokies. I was trying to get some sourwood blossoms for my wife to press and add to her collection when I got stung by a bee. It was in the blossoms, and I didn't even see it. I guess it was so busy trying to get sourwood nectar that it didn't see me either. Anyway, I got stung on the hand. First sting I've had in a long time too. My hand swelled up, and my arm almost to the shoulder. I felt kind of funny, like this last time. Weak and dizzy and sort of, well, choked up. It all passed pretty quickly. I meant to ask you next time we played tennis. You remember, I beat you pretty badly. You claimed it was an off day or some such rot. You were so upset that I hadn't the heart to burden you with my troubles. Then I forgot.

Of course, my friend had had a systemic reaction from the bee sting up there in the Great Smokies. The next time around he almost lost his life. The Great Smoky Mountains bee had increased his sensitivity so that the bees at home almost did him in. The moral of the tale is that, if you suffer any of the symptoms of generalized systemic reaction following a bee-sting (or the sting or bite of any other insect), consult your physician at once. Not next month or next year, but next day.

The Hazard of Bees

Do not put it off. Badger the doctor on the tennis court if you must, but apprize him of your problem. He wants to know, for the next time you get stung could be your last. There is always a good chance that you might not make it to the emergency room in time. Time, as we have noted, is all too often something that individuals allergic to insect venom do not have. For the next chapter we will assume that the reader—an intelligent, careful person in love with his life—does consult his doctor, and we will see what methods of treatment bee and other stings call for and how one can, insofar as is humanly possible, protect oneself.

READER'S GUIDE TO ALLERGIC REACTION

The symptoms:

Normal reaction to an insect sting or bite:
Momentary pain; redness around the bite or sting site, surrounded by a whitish zone or a hivelike red spot; itching; irritation; and heat. All traces are usually gone within a few hours.

Local reaction to a sting or bite:
More than the normal amount of swelling, pain, and redness at the bite site. Symptoms usually vanish within a few hours.

Allergic, or generalized systemic, reaction to a sting or bite:

- First-degree symptoms:
  Itching around the eyes, dry hacking cough, widespread hives, constriction of chest and throat, wheezing, nausea, abdominal pain, vomiting, dizziness.
- More severe symptoms:
  Difficulty in breathing, hoarseness and thickened speech, difficulty in swallowing, confusion, a sense of impending disaster.

57

- Anaphylactic shock symptoms:
  Cyanosis, reduced blood pressure, collapse, incontinence, unconsciousness.

Toxic reaction to multiple stings or bites:
Headache, diarrhea, faintness, fever, drowsiness, swelling, unconsciousness, convulsions.

Delayed reaction to stings or bites:
Headache, malaise, hives, aching joints, lymph involvement.

Psychological reaction to stings or bites:
Rapid heartbeat; rapid, shallow breathing; weakness; dizziness.

When to consult a doctor:

- When a local reaction exhibits undue swelling covering two joints of a leg, arm, or hand or when a sting causes swelling in the throat, nose, or eye, particularly the latter. A sting close to the eye should be seen by a doctor because complications can result that threaten sight.
- When a sting results in symptoms of a generalized systemic reaction, no matter how mild.
- When multiple stings produce signs of a toxic reaction.
- When the swelling accompanying a normal or local reaction persists, because infection may have set in.
- When symptoms of a delayed reaction appear.

5

Insect-Sting Treatment and Prevention

A child comes running into the house, streaming tears, one hand held high, or hopping on one leg. crying. "Mommy, Mommy, I been hurted!" A man mowing his lawn suddenly swats wildly at the air around his head, drops his mower, and runs. A woman reaches for a cucumber dangling on the vine, but backs off with a little shriek of pain. All over the land during the summer months scenes like these occur. The stingers are out in full force.

What do you do if you are the central character in such a scenario? While we are focusing on beestings at the moment, the treatment for the stings of wasps, yellow jackets, and hornets—which we will discuss in the next chapter—is the same. We should note also that the person allergic to the sting of one member of the Hymenoptera clan is often allergic to the venom of several members. Thus the person allergic to beestings may well be allergic to the stings of wasps or yellow jackets or hornets or ants or all of those. This is called *cross-reactivity*, and it is thought to result from sensitivity to some common factor or constituent in the venom of the various stingers.

Many asthma and allergic-rhinitis patients are also allergic to insects, as are frequently those who have a family history of allergy. Almost one third of the patients allergic to insect stings are also allergic to drugs, particularly those that are injected, and particularly penicillin. Thus there are certain individuals who, when they have been the central character in one of our little scenarios, should be especially wary. They are the ones who may need to seek medical aid.

But here you are, a little angry, a little shocked by the suddenness of the attack, a little distressed by the sharp pin-prick of pain. The bee has struggled away to die, leaving her stinger in your flesh. The attached venom sac is still pulsing, still pumping venom into your skin. What do you do? Do not seize the stinger to remove it, for this will simply force more venom into the wound. Rather, scrape it out with your fingernail or a knife. Then follow the cardinal rule for all insect stings or bites: wash the area well with soap and water. Secondary infection can cause far more trouble than a normal reaction to such attacks. Once well washed, ice packs will relieve the pain and reduce the subsequent swelling. The old home remedy of a paste of baking soda mixed with a little water also relieves pain. In any case, if the reaction is normal, you will probably forget the whole episode in an hour or so, although you may be a bit more wary of the insect world than formerly.

Treatment for a normal or a mild local reaction is relatively simple. It consists of relieving the pain and minimizing the chances of secondary infection in the sting wound. When there is a severe local reaction, with considerable swelling and hardening of the flesh around the sting site, the above measures should also be taken, with the addition of rest and elevation of the limb if an arm or leg is involved. Exercise will only increase the swelling and make it last longer. If the swelling is such that it covers two joints of an extremity, or if it is in the throat, nose, or eye area, a doctor should be consulted, as we stated in the preceding chapter. Antihistamines may help control some of the swelling and will relieve subsequent itching. On occasion, if the swelling is protracted and resists everyday measures, steroids are used.

When there are symptoms of a generalized systemic reaction, we must remember that even the mildest of signs may become an emergency matter within minutes. Thus it is important to seek medical help at the first sign of an allergic reaction. The stinger should be scraped out at once, and ice packs applied to slow the absorption of the venom. If the sting is on a limb, a tourniquet will help to slow the spread of the venom, but it must be loosened frequently, at least every three to five minutes. I repeat, however, that the most important thing to do is to get the victim to the nearest doctor or hospital emergency room as quickly as possible.

What kind of measures are taken to relieve systemic symptoms? Most important, in order to abort anaphylactic shock reactions, is an immediate injection of epinephrine (adrenaline), to be followed in fifteen or twenty minutes by a second injection if symptoms are not relieved. In the meantime antihistamines may be injected intramuscularly, oxygen may be administered if the patient has become cyanotic, and other measures may be taken to support blood pressure and circulation. It is the epinephrine, however, that is vital. It is the one measure upon which the insect-allergic individual's life depends when he suffers a severe systemic reaction. Because this is so, I have mounted a white horse to advocate that insect-sting kits containing preloaded syringes of epinephrine be placed wherever the public may encounter Hymenoptera and be stung by them. Boy-Scout and Girl-Scout leaders, forest rangers, lifeguards, golf and tennis pros, school nurses, and the like should not only have these kits handy but also be familiar with their contents and their use. Legislation should allow the use of such kits by nonmedical personnel in emergency situations.

An insect-sting kit, like a snakebite kit, is compact and portable. It contains the syringe preloaded with the proper amount of epinephrine, a tourniquet, several antihistamine tablets to be taken orally, several sterilizing alcohol pads, and often several tranquilizers. Simple, clear instructions accompany the kit. But it is not designed to replace prompt medical aid. It is still vital to get the victim to a hospital or a physician as quickly as possible. The kit is meant to stave off the fulminating symptoms long enough for the victim to get to that hospital or physician. A good many insect-sting victims suffer their attacks many miles and minutes from a medical facility. Sometimes they are hours away, and as we have seen, severe systemic reactions can be fatal within ten or fifteen minutes, often within the first half hour, after a sting. In fact, if the victim of a systemic reaction to insect venom survives the first hour, he is usually out of the woods. Commonly, the more rapidly the initial systemic symptoms develop the greater chances are of fatality.

In most, if not all, of the United States the insect-sting kit must be prescribed by a physician. It is not an over-the-counter item. Any person who has suffered even mild symptoms of a systemic reaction as described in **Appendix A**, or even just a severe local reaction, should request a prescription for a kit (or several kits) from their doctor. They should keep a kit handy wherever there is a chance of being stung. Incidentally, if the epinephrine in the syringe turns brown, it should be immediately replaced. The kits will soon contain a more stable form of epinephrine, which the manufacturers say will remain good for three years.

A further recommendation of all those who have suffered insect-allergic symptoms is that they wear a medical warning tag or bracelet to alert medical personnel of their allergy in case they lose consciousness or coherence. Many an insect-sting victim has gone unrecognized because sting wounds are small and often go unnoticed. Precious time may be lost as the physician tries to decide whether the patient is suffering from heat stroke, heart attack, or some other illness. See **Appendix C** for more information about such tags.

Once the emergency of a severe generalized systemic reaction is over, the patient and his physician must think of long-term management of the problem. There is always the chance of being restung and the ever-present possibility that the next sting will produce even more severe symptoms. Measures to protect the victim and prevent future attacks now become important.

The *hyposensitization, or desensitization, procedure* should be started at once. In this procedure the allergic person's tolerance to insect venom is raised by injections of extracts of ground-up whole bodies of the offending insects or, as of recently, injections of extracts of insect venom. Initial injections are exceedingly weak. Gradually the strength of the extracts is increased over time until the patient can tolerate what might be a normal exposure to insect or beestings. At that point the patient is kept on a maintenance dose to keep his tolerance high. The procedure is really an immunization, and it is generally very effective. Approximately 97 percent of the patients who arrive at a maintenance dose have less-severe allergic reactions to subsequent stings. At one time it was thought that the patient would have adequate protection if he remained on a maintenance dose for three years. However, when failure began to appear occasionally, the term was extended to ten years. As of this writing we really do not know how long a patient should be kept on a maintenance dose. My patients stay on such injections indefinitely. It may sound like a terrible nuisance (and expense) to roll up one's sleeve and present one's arm to the nurse and her needle every seven days during Hymenoptera season (from April to October throughout much of the country and from April to December in my native South) and every two to three weeks thereafter, but this is the only way that those who are allergic can go in safety and with peace of mind.

After reaching a maintenance dose and after being restung without any reaction, patients sometimes arrived triumphantly in my office to proclaim that they have bested the bee and so, "Good-bye, Dr. Frazier!" They have gone their merry way only to return chastened and a little scared after being stung once again some time later with a return of systemic symptoms. The maintenance dose lives up to its name: it maintains tolerance levels. And safe is always better than sorry.

In medicine, as in just about everything else in life, nothing is 100 percent certain. Therefore, I prescribe an insect-sting kit as a matter of course for my insect-allergic patients. In fact, I prescribe several—one for home, one for car, and so on. And I badger the patients off and on to make sure they do not become too complacent.

In an informal survey that I made recently fifteen physicians wrote me that they were unaware of the kit's existence, and only four wrote that they knew about it. Among laymen allergic to insects, only one wrote that he knew about the kit, while ten did not. Of all the patients I have seen in my office who have had severe systemic reactions to insect stings, eight out of ten do not possess the kit and never had a kit prescribed by the physicians who treated their reactions. Some of those patients suffered severe reactions two or three years before I saw them. They were walking about as endangered as if they carried time bombs in their pockets, especially during the early months of hyposensitization when they were still quite vulnerable.

It is not easy to make believers of either patients or physicians. We large, and generally hardy, human beings find it difficult to comprehend that anything as small as a bee can kill us. For instance, not long ago I gave a talk on insect allergy at a medical meeting. A physician approached me later to tell me in tones of disbelief of a recent case of his. The patient in question was a farmer who was stung while plowing in his field. His wife heard him yell, "I've been stung!," but before she could get to him, he was dead. According to his wife, he had been stung previously and had suffered symptoms of a systemic reaction. The colleague who told me this had not believed that a person could die from an insect sting, and he recorded the farmer's death on the certificate as "due to heart attack."

We need to make believers of our lawmakers also if we are to prevent needless tragedies. For example, I had a young patient not long ago who had a very close call with a beesting. I recommended that the parents apprize the school authorities of the future danger, especially until we could get the youngster to a maintenance dose in his desensitization treatment, and I recommended that they supply an insect-sting kit to the school nurse in case the child was restung during school. The parents were informed that, even if the nurse had the kit, she could not legally give an injection without the express orders of a physician called on the case. "The best we can do," the school officials said, "is call an ambulance or have the child driven to the hospital or doctor's office." Both the nearest hospital and the nearest physician's office were more than a half hour away.

Can the allergic individual prevent being stung in the first place? That is a good question. No one, I suppose, can be a 100 percent sure of avoiding the attentions of a bee, whether a honeybee, humblebee, or even the far gentler sweat bee. Certainly, though, there are steps one can take to minimize the chances of collision. They are listed in the reader's guide at the end of this chapter and again in **Appendix E.** Such measures should help the allergic individual to "bee" prepared not only against chance attacks from bees but also against encounters with other members of the order Hymenoptera, such as wasps, yellow jackets, hornets, and even ants, as we shall see in the chapters that follow.

READER'S GUIDE TO TREATMENT AND PREVENTION

What to do if stung by a bee:

Home treatment:

- Scrape out the stinger, if one is present, with fingernail or knife (bumblebee stingers do not have barbs and are not left in the wound).
- Wash the sting site well with soap and water.
- Apply an ice pack and/or a paste of baking soda and water to relieve pain.
- Be alert for symptoms of systemic reaction or unusual swelling, especially swelling that extends far beyond the sting site.

Emergency treatment for allergic, or systemic, reaction:

- Remove the stinger and use an insect-sting kit as directed if one is obtainable; then rush the victim to the nearest doctor or hospital.
- If an insect-sting kit is unobtainable, remove the stinger, apply an ice pack if possible, and rush the victim to the nearest doctor or hospital.

What to expect in long-term management of insect-sting allergy:

- Immediate initiation of the hyposensitization procedure.
- Prescription for the insect-sting kit with careful instructions on its use.
- Recommendation to wear a warning tag or bracelet.

How to keep from being stung:

- Stay away from beehives and known nests. Call a beekeeper or the fire department if bees choose your immediate environment to form a colony.
- Persons allergic to insects should be wary of power mowing, hedge clipping, scything, and the like.
- Avoid looking and smelling like a flower during Hymenoptera season: avoid bright-colored clothing, foreswear perfumes and sweet smelling lotions, creams, shampoos, and the like.
- Do not wear floppy clothing, and do tie up long hair, for both can entangle the stinging insects and anger them into doing their worst.
- Do not go barefoot or wear sandals—the foot is vulnerable. Stay away from clover patches, flower gardens, and other places where bees are busy. Let someone else pick the flowers.
- Wear light-colored clothing during the warm months: light green, white, tan, and khaki are safest.

Sting Treatment and Prevention

- Keep an insecticide spray in the glove compartment of the car (along with the insect-sting kit) for use if a bee flies in, a very common occurrence.
- If an attack seems imminent, do not swat at the bee or bees and do not flail your arms. Retreat slowly, keep calm, and make no sudden movement. If retreat is impossible, lie down and cover your head with your arms.

6

Wasps, Hornets, and Yellow Jackets

A woman in her mid-sixties was fishing from a boat on our large lake. She and her husband were sharing a can of beer on the seat between them, each taking a sip now and then. Finally the can was about gone, so she took the last swallow and immediately experienced severe pain in the upper chest and then in the lower chest. [She] felt miserable for a few minutes and soon began to vomit. Apparently she also felt weak.

"She vomited into a bucket and up came a yellow jacket—by this time dead, of course. She then felt better and as they were quite a way out in the lake, they continued fishing.

The doctor who wrote me about this case went on to say that all was well with the lady who swallowed a yellow jacket in her beer, although internal stings are surely the exception rather than the rule and certainly are uncomfortable. I cite the case, however, to illustrate that the stingers are apt to be anywhere and everywhere and especially where you least expect to find them.

More cases of beestings are actually documented than of stings of wasps, hornets, or yellow jackets, but the latter three are more aggressive than bees, with the exception, of course, of the killer bees of Africa and Brazil. You do not come away unscathed after innocently bumping into wasp, hornet, or yellow-jacket nests. In fact, your very approach may bring them out in a swarm. Vibrations from a tractor or mower, for

68

instance, will bring forth yellow jackets who are nesting in the ground nearby, ready for battle. In fact, it is the social members of the order of Hymenoptera, rather than the solitary, who generally do the stinging, perhaps because the solitary bee or wasp recognizes that one small insect alone can do little damage. The solitary mud-dauber wasps, for instance, who plaster their nests under the eaves, rarely sting; and when they do, their venom usually causes a mild allergic reaction if any.

Wasps, hornets, and yellow jackets belong to the social vespid family of Hymenoptera. One of the more interesting of the solitary wasps is the velvet ant, more popularly called the cow killer because of its potent sting. The female is noticeable because she is wingless and runs about on the ground much like a large ant. Velvet ants are often large and brightly colored, and it is their habit to seek out the nests of other solitary wasps or bees, which the hardworking owner has stocked with provisions for its own larvae. The velvet ant will lay its egg amid the goodies, and because its egg will hatch first, the newcomer will not only finish off the provisions but the owner's young as well.

The majority of solitary hunting wasps lay their eggs in insects, such as caterpillars, that they have paralyzed or killed. Thus the hatching larvae have ready-made meals close to hand. Some simply leave both caterpillar and egg where they chanced to be; others will cart the caterpillar back to a nest to give their developing larvae some protection. One hunting wasp in the Southwest, called the tarantula killer, has developed her predation to an exquisite art. She will go down a tarantula's burrow to tangle with it on its own home territory. She somehow entices the tarantula to rear back on its hand legs and expose its vulnerable underbelly to her stinger. Her venom paralyzes the far-larger insect and preserves it for her larder for as long as thirty-five to forty days.

Adult solitary wasps commonly dine on nectar and juices of fruits, but they spend a good part of their lives collecting other insects to feed their young. The larvae of the different species seem to have decided preferences for this or that kind of insect, preferring, for instance, spiders to caterpillars or flies to tarantulas. Entomologists, who likewise spend a good part of their time collecting insects, know that the nests of solitary wasps are often rich lodes containing various species difficult to locate elsewhere. One scientist working in the Congo found over two hundred different species of flies in the nests of solitary wasps, some of which have not been seen anywhere since, presumably because they are elusive to man, although not to hunting wasps.

The two solitary wasps most familiar in our land are the digger and the mud dauber. Digger wasps are especially interesting because they use a tool, a pebble, in the construction of their nests. Observers report that the wasp picks up a small pebble in its jaws to hammer the dirt over its nest, drops the pebble to gather more dirt, then picks up the pebble to hammer some more. The digger larvae prefer caterpillars as food, so the female paralyzes a goodly supply, transports them to the nest, and leaves her eggs sealed in among the helpless, hapless caterpillars.

Anyone who has ever broken into a mud dauber's nest on a wall is startled at the number of spiders, flies, and the like that come tumbling out. The nest, made of mud and tiny pebbles, is usually located on a sunny wall or rock face and consists of a number of cells arranged in an elongated row. When the first cell is constructed and filled with eggs, another cell is built, and so on. Papa dauber often stands guard during the process while the female goes off for mud or provisions.

Fly-catching wasps do a great favor to man and, in the case of "horse guards," to livestock. One single fly-catching wasp ate eighty-two flies within eight days, a regimen that would certainly take care of the fly population if only enough of the wasps would hang around. These sand, or Bembecid, wasps are semisocial. The females often make their burrows close together, although each goes her own way in life.

Our main problems with wasps come from the social variety—the Polistes wasp, the hornet, and the yellow jacket. They can be the nemesis of the allergic and nonallergic alike.

Wasps, Hornets, and Yellow Jackets

The Polistes wasp is found almost everywhere in the world, including Europe and our own country, where it is familiarly known as the paper wasp. These wasps find their way into our attics when the first cold days of fall arrive. Mercifully, they are not particularly aggressive and will leave us alone, given the chance. They will sting upon provocation, however, and their sting can be painful. Although potent for the allergic, their venom is not as bad as that of their cousins the yellow jackets and hornets. They make their flat, open-celled nests in sheltered spots, such as under the eaves of barns and houses. The material, or "paper," is made of wood chewed to a pulp. The nests are not as large as those constructed by either the yellow jackets or the hornets.

The eggs are cemented to the roof of the cells, one egg to each cell, and when the larvae emerge, a strange exchange of favors takes place. The queens and worker wasps hasten to catch and chew up caterpillars and other choice insect tidbits, then feed them to the larvae, who hang head down, at the ready, so to speak. In exchange the larvae are expected to produce a delicious drop of saliva, which is greedily sucked up by the adult wasp. If the drop is not forthcoming, the stubborn larva is prodded until it gives it out. Sometimes it is prodded to produce even when no mushed-up caterpillar or the like is offered in exchange, and sometimes it is prodded so frequently and must give so generously that it becomes malnourished and stunted. It is thought that this is what causes some wasps to be sterile workers and that they are thereafter kept sterile because of all the hard work they do building the nest and hunting provisions. The mutual exchange of delicacies is called trophallaxis, a word derived from the Greek word *trophi* meaning to feed. It is thought that this mutual nutritional dependence is what brought the wasps together in the first place and kept them social. Toward the end of summer, perhaps because food is far more abundant, the larvae do better nutritionally and become fully sexed. Earlier in the season the queen has gathered all her sperm as the flowers of May and kept them in a separate sac in her abdomen. In the fall she chooses not to fertilize some of the eggs she lays, and these unfertilized eggs develop into males, who in turn fill the sperm sacs of young queens.

When the cold of autumn draws near, fewer and fewer workers are produced; the original queen, now ancient, ceases her egg laying; and the colony dissipates. Only the young queens survive; only those, that is, who can find shelter from the winter cold in warm places such as our attics. In the spring they reactivate from their state of hibernation to fly off to found new colonies and begin the process all over again. Probably only a few of many survive, but apparently enough to keep the Polistes going.

As some of us are unhappily aware, hornets and yellow jackets build far larger nests than do Polistes wasps—in holes in the ground, in rotton logs or posts, or hanging from trees or bushes. As often as not we find them the hard way be bumping against them or stepping into them. The resulting swarm of angry, aggressive stingers is both horrifying and impressive. The nests start small with a single tier of cells, but the busy efforts of the inhabitants soon add another and another until the colony becomes quite formidable. Above ground, nests are encased in a tough sheath. As the nest enlarges the outer wraps are torn down and rebuilt to accommodate the growing nest. There can be as many as five thousand lively hornets or yellow jackets in one such nest.

As the eggs hatch, the queen who started it all feeds the initial larvae. Because she must do this on her own, the first individuals that emerge are smaller than the later arrivals, whom they help to feed. Once the colony has arrived at an optimum size, there is a division of labor of a sort among the workers. Some hunt for food; some stay home to feed the larvae, add to the cell tiers, guard the entrance to the nest, and even ventilate the home by fanning their wings. Toward the end of summer, it is thought, some of the workers that are not wholly sterile lay unfertilized eggs, which produce males who in turn will fertilize the young queens. As with the Polistes, some of the young queens will survive the winter to begin new colonies in the spring. And the males? Well, their duty done, they quickly die.

Adult hornets and yellow jackets prefer fruit juices, nectar, and fermenting sap to eat, but they are fierce predators, capturing a variety of insects to mush up for their larvae. They are also scavengers and can be found in swarms around decomposing animal flesh, which must be taken into consideration in the treatment of their stings. Secondary infection is a far likelier contingency from their attack than from the sting of a bee.

On the plus side of the ledger, yellow jackets and hornets cross-pollinate flowers, crops, and fruit, although they are not as prodigious in these helpful efforts as are the bees. If only they would stay out in the wild. Unfortunately, they have an affinity for the works of man, preferring to build their nests in his lampposts and fence posts, along his walls, and under his steps, porches, and eaves. It is the misfortune of both hornets and small boys that the hornets' football-sized nests present an almost irresistable temptation to the casting of stones. I have had any number of young fellows in my office who were unable to pass up such an attraction. To them I say, "He who casts upon paper houses is likely to get stung."

As a matter of fact, we can even construct a model of the kind of youngster who is likely to get stung by one or the other or all of the species of Hymenoptera discussed here. The sting-prone child is a boy somewhere between the ages of five and eight. He is energetic and curious and likes to chase things that run or fly. He is barefoot and bareheaded, and the yard he usually plays in is loaded with clover and decorated by flower beds. His mother dresses him in bright-colored shirts, and in earlier decades she might douse his unruly hair with hair oil. He is not one to look before he leaps.

The stings of wasps, hornets, and yellow jackets can be a very serious business. Their venom, like the venom of bees, can cause severe allergic reactions in the sensitive and even fatalities. Not long ago a brief account in a Tennessee newspaper told of a man who lifted a bale of hay near his home under which yellow jackets were nesting. Stung, he collapsed and died almost immediately. A good deal of reasearch has been done recently to sort out the components of Hymenoptera venom. If we knew exactly what chemical substance caused allergic and toxic effects in sting victims, we would have come a long way in our efforts to counter such effects. So far the most that can be said is that no one single substance is the apparent cause of the reaction; rather it is the combined action of a number of chemicals contained in the venom. One constituent, which is also found in snake venom, destroys red blood cells; another lowers blood pressure; still another affects the nervous system. All in all, even though the amount of venom injected per sting is very small, the substances it contains are exceedingly potent.

An interesting case was reported recently in the *Journal of the American Medical Association*. Twenty-four hours after being stung by wasps a man developed symptoms of myasthenia gravis, a disease in which the muscles progressively weaken. The onset of this serious disease is usually gradual, beginning with drooping of the eyelids and difficulty in chewing and swallowing. The man in question had enjoyed excellent health until stung on the finger by three Polistes wasps. His whole hand became swollen and reddened. Shortly after he was stung, his left eyelid began to droop. A few days later the right side of his forehead and his right ear became markedly swollen. After the swelling of his face subsided, the eyelid continued to droop, and the right eyelid also began to give him trouble. Within a few months tests were made, and myasthenia gravis diagnosed.

Involvement of the central nervous system is somewhat less common than other effects of venom, but in one hundred fatal cases, seven were due to such factors. Most such reactions occur several days after the sting. There is one case on record that connects personality change, abnormal behavior, and permanent mental confusion and disorientation to the sting of a bee. Hymenoptera venom can cause neuritis, or inflammation of the nerves, with resulting muscular disorders, including clumsiness, weakness, numbness, tingling, and prickling in an affected extremity. One woman patient, stung on a finger of her left hand, still felt such effects in her hand and wrist seven months later.

One possible result of a sting by a wasp, hornet, or yellow jacket, especially the latter, is the transmission of infection to the wound, since as we mentioned earlier, these members of the Hymenoptera clan, unlike bees, are scavengers and are likely to have been rummaging about in decaying carcasses, among other things. Because the sting is a puncture wound, the infection can take the form of cellulitis, a severe inflammation of the tissues, which needs immediate treatment by a doctor. Symptoms are swelling, heat in the area, redness, and pain.

Thus the venomous vespids can be vicious.

READER'S GUIDE TO WASPS, HORNETS, AND YELLOW JACKETS

Know the enemy:

The polistes wasp:
   Usually reddish brown in color, it is slender with a spindle-shaped abdomen. **(See Plates 4 and 5.)** Its nest consists of a single tier of cells, is more or less circular in appearance, and is attached by a thin stalk, often under barn and house eaves.

The yellow jacket:
   Smaller than a wasp, it has black and yellow stripes much like those of a hornet. **(See Plates 6 and 7.)** Its nest consists of several tiers of cells and is often to be found in old posts, stumps, and holes in the ground

The hornet:
   The most familiar species is large and black with yellowish-white markings. **(See Plates 8 and 9.)** The nests are large and football-shaped and commonly hang from the branches of a tree or bush, although sometimes they are built in grass.

WASPS, HORNETS, AND YELLOW JACKETS

What to do if stung:

Home treatment:
- Wasps, yellow jackets, and hornets leave no stinger in the wound since their stingers are not barbed.
- Wash the sting area well with soap and water. This is vital because these insects are scavengers, and secondary infection is a very real possibility.
- Apply an ice pack and/or a paste of baking soda and water.
- Be alert for allergic reaction symptoms or more-than-usual swelling.

Emergency treatment for allergic reaction:
- Use the insect-sting kit as directed, if one is available, and rush the victim to the nearest physician or hospital.
- If no insect-sting kit is available, apply an ice pack if possible, and rush the victim to the nearest physician or hospital.

What should be done in long-term management of allergy to vespid stings:

- Immediate initiation of the hyposensitization procedure.
- Prescription for an insect-sting kit with careful instructions in its use and with a warning to keep it at hand whenever and wherever Hymenoptera may be encountered (it is best to have several kits).
- Recommendation that the victim wear a warning tag or bracelet.

How to keep from being stung:

- Have wasp, yellow-jacket, and hornet nests removed while they are still small enough to handle. Wasp nests can be knocked from walls or from under eaves with a broom handle or may be hosed off (but not by the allergic individual). The area should be sprayed with an insecticide to discourage rebuilding. Yellow-jacket nests in the ground should be marked during the day; then gas, kerosine, lye, or an insecticide should be poured or sprayed into the hole at night. Lighting the gas or kerosine is not necessary; the fumes will do the trick. Repeat the procedure the following night. Hornet nests should be removed by a professional exterminator or the fire department. Make periodic searches for such nests in the home and yard from early spring until the first frosts. In the fall check the attic for wasps that have come to hibernate.

- If allergic, do not mow, clip hedges, prune trees, scythe tall grass, and the like.
- Keep an aerosol insecticide and insect-sting kit in the glove compartment of the car if wasps or other stinging insects are likely to fly in.
- Wear khaki, white, tan, or light-green clothing during the summer months rather than bright colors, and do not use scented products on the body when you are going to be outdoors.
- Do not go barefoot or wear sandals.
- Do not wear floppy clothing that may entangle these notoriously bad-tempered stingers, and keep long hair tied up. Keep skin exposure to a minimum wherever Hymenoptera may be encountered.
- If apparently about to be attacked, do not swat or flail your arms. Retreat slowly, keep calm, and make no sudden movements. If retreat seems impossible, lie flat and cover your head with your arms.
- Discourage allergic youngsters from consuming sweets such as Popsicles, ice-cream cones, and soda pop outdoors during the warm months.
- Be wary in the vicinity of garbage cans, rotting fruit under trees, and the like because they attract yellow jackets and wasps (as well as bees).

7

If Allergic,
Do Not Go to the Ant

The ghost of a great green ant sits astride one of the richest uranium-ore deposits in the world, and all the men of a mining company have so far been unable to change the aborigines' refusal to sell the mining rights to the find. They will not sell because green ants live in an area near the lode, and where the green ants live is hallowed ground. The aborigine legend says that, if they are disturbed, the ants will turn into man-eating monsters, so voracious that they will destroy the world. Never mind that it is the uranium beneath the ants' stamping ground that is most likely to finish off mother earth, the green ants must not be bothered. So far the aborigines have refused all sorts of financial blandishments. Money versus monsters is no contest.

There are about fifteen thousand different ant species, although to the untutored eye there may appear to be simply big ants and little ants, red ants, black ants, and of course, green ants. Ants, like their Hymenoptera cousins the bees, are hardworking and highly organized. They have moved so successfully down the corridors of time few places on earth have managed to stay free of their presence. Ants do many things well: nest building, scavengering for food, slave making, society organizing, and propagating their own kind. The last is probably what they do best, as anyone can testify who has seen an anthill spring up practically overnight on the lawn. The sex life of an ant is geared to colonizing the country-side. Hundreds, sometimes thousands, of winged males and females will leave an established ant colony to begin hun-dreds, sometimes thousands, of new colonies, for the young queens are accompanied on their marriage flight by their lov-ers, who die when the flight is over. The queens, fecund by the time they land, remove their wings by rubbing or chewing them off and retreat, each alone, to a suitable spot to lay their first batches of eggs. Sometimes they find an ideal spot in broken soil, sometimes in a crevice or behind loose bark on a tree. In any case, wherever the lady chooses, she lays a few eggs. She tends the resulting larvae by herself, using her now-useless wing muscles for her own nourishment and for the production of the salivary secretions that she feeds to her larvae. Some kinds of ants vary this theme. In some species the female carries a few worker ants on her marriage flight to help her out with the nursery chores later. They cling to her legs as she and the male consummate their nuptials, then land with her as her maids-in-waiting.

The first batch of larvae are females, but because mother has not much to feed them, they are undernourished, sterile, and stunted. Even though they are puny, they take over the work of the colony, and the queen is free to keep on laying eggs, for her a lifetime chore. She apparently has the choice of who and what her offspring will be. She possesses a sperm sac, which was filled on her marriage flight by her now-defunct lover. She seems to be able to fertilize some eggs and not others. Those that she fertilizes hatch out as new queens, workers, or soldiers. Those that she chooses not to fertilize and those that she lays after the sperm sac has been depleted turn out to be the unfortunate males. Of course, whether this is really choice or random chance is anyone's guess, but it does work out that most of her eggs are fertilized, and just enough eggs are left unfertilized so that the species will pro-duce sufficient males to fertilize the young queens. It takes four or five years generally for the colony to produce indi-viduals sufficiently well nourished to become queens and males. Thus ants do not swarm too frequently, and that one anthill on the lawn has to be there for a while before the others will spring up seemingly overnight.

Ants are long-lived, remarkably so for insects, many of whom die within a few days or weeks after reaching adulthood. Ant queens have been known to reach the hoary age of twenty, and workers live around ten years. Such advanced ages were achieved, however, among captives. Ants in the wild probably fall victim to predators or are stepped on long before they can attain such an age. Research has shown, though, that the elderly ants in a colony give the younger ants the benefit of their hard-won experience, which may well be one reason ants have been so successful. Often such an elderly, experienced ant is the one who initiates ant activity and acts as the leader whom the rest of the ants follow. When she moves off to hunt for food, the other workers follow. A winter of hibernation does not appear to dim the older ant's "memory" of food areas and ant paths used the year before.

An ant's sense of taste and smell is acute. Its sight is much dimmer, and some kinds of ants do not see at all. Ants constantly groom each other, imparting the colony odor. Any intruder without the proper smell is immediately kicked out or killed, but if the stranger can somehow remain long enough to take on the colony's very special scent, it will be accepted. If she smells like every other ant in the heap, she belongs; if she does not, she is harried from the hill. Even dead ants are licked and groomed, apparently until their scent wears off or is stifled by the smell of decomposition. Once this happens, the corpse is hastily bundled out of the nest. In an interesting experiment a researcher daubed living ants with the smell of decomposition. As soon as the unfortunates entered the nest they were hustled back outside by the workers. When they struggled back in again, they were once more dumped beyond the entrance. This went on until the smell of decomposition evidently wore off. Only then were they allowed to make it back into the anthill to resume their duties.

Anyone who has broken into an anthill and observed the

contents knows that it contains dozens, sometimes hundreds, of tiny white larvae and that the ants will pick these up immediately and scurry madly in their efforts to take their progeny to safety. Initially the larvae are not much more than a mouth. After a few days spent at this odd stage, they become pupae, which remain immobile and foodless until they emerge as mature ants.

The food habits of ants are strange and interesting. Most of us are aware that ants have a relationship to aphids much as we do to dairy cows. Aphids suck sap from plants, and when stroked by their ant "owner," they secrete a drop of honeydew, which is evidently an ant delight. In return, the ants protect the aphids. If they are threatened, the ant will do battle for them or even pick up the endangered aphid and try to carry it to safety as they do their own larvae. Some ants build shelters for their aphid herds on the stems that are their pastures, and some will pick up the aphids and carry them to new plants when the pasturage grows lean. In the winter they carry aphid eggs into their underground nests to give them the best of care, thus ensuring next year's honeydew. Some ants maintain a similar relationship with several types of caterpillars that also produce honeydew.

A remarkable kind of ant actually practices farming by raising fungi on a pulp they make of chewed-up leaves. They gather the leaves, manufacture the pulp, and store it in a storehouse, where, as it decays, it grows a crop of ant mushrooms. Not only that. The young queens carry a pellet of fungi as a starter for the new colony that they will found. Before they go off on their marriage flight, they pick up their bit of starter, and when they lay their first batch of eggs, the fungi are stored nearby. The fungi are fertilized by the ant's droppings so that, by the time the larvae appear, food is on the table.

Of all ant dietary delights, honeydew appears to take the cake—or rather be the cake. Certain honey ants store this delicacy in a most unusual manner. Some young ants are selected, or elected, to be honeydew pots. They are filled to capacity with the honey. Unable to move because of their enforced obesity, they hang from the ceiling of the nest and give forth of their contents to their hungry comrades upon demand. They spend their entire life hanging there by their feet, discharging honeydew when properly stroked, an ant version of a vending machine.

Many ant species communicate by leaving scent trails. These chemical secretions are celled pheromones. It is believed that there are many different such scents—some to attract, others to repel, and some even to sound the alarm. Like the dance of the bee on the threshold of the hive, the chemical trails lead to food areas. Hundreds of ants will scurry back and forth along the trails, for all the world like traffic on an interstate. They will respond like robots to the particular pheromone transmitted by their fellows, but mysteriously one kind of ant will pay no attention to the pheromone of a different species. This is fortunate, since many ant species will inhabit a given area. It is easy to imagine what would happen if the different species got their trails crossed.

Slavery is another strange institution of some ant species. These species will conduct regular raids on the nests of other ants and scatter the enemy's workers. Then they will seize the larvae and pupae and take them back to their own nests, where they raise them as workers. Unlike human slaves, however, the slaves apparently become equal members of the colony of their captors. The amazon ants are the strangest of all the slave makers, for they apparently are physically and mentally unable to do for themselves and can survive only by the efforts of their slaves. They will even starve to death with food aplenty heaped about them if a slave is not around to feed it to them.

Ants are everywhere. Sometimes this is fortunate for us and sometimes unfortunate. Like earthworms, ants aerate the soil and make it pervious to water, and they prey upon many insects that are harmful to human crops and livestock. Unfortunately, they also cultivate the aphid, which attacks our cultivated crops, and leaf-cutting ants by themselves can do a great deal of harm. The two ants that are directly harmful to human health in our own land are the red harvester and the fire ant. Both are stingers capable of producing fatal toxic or allergic reactions. The two species are widespread throughout the southern and western United States. Their venom can cause severe reactions in hypersensitive individuals and can do the nonallergic a bit of damage also.

Harvester ants, which may be black or red in color, have a vicious sting and are quite aggressive. Their nests are large, low mounds that can denude an extensive area of vegetation as they increase in size. The harvesters acquired their name from their habit of gathering seeds and storing them in their hills. The seeds that they drop about the entrance to the colony often sprout, and the resulting crops of weeds were mistaken in the past for a cultivated patch deliberately sown by the ants, although they are apparently just the results of carelessness. There are cases on record of small animals blundering into red-harvester anthills and being stung to death, but the mounds are distinctive, and fortunately, few human beings have ventured into them. A harvester ant's sting can be very painful, and they can cause severe systemic reactions.

But the real ant villain, as far as we are concerned, is the fire ant, especially the imported variety. The imported fire ant has received a good deal of notoriety in recent years because of the extensive damage it has inflicted on southern crop and pasture lands. Our own domestic fire ant is not guiltless, but the hitchhiker from South America, who arrived on our shores some fifty years ago, has been amazingly fecund. First seen in Mobile, Alabama, where, it is thought, it arrived by ship, the imported fire ant has spread over about ten or twelve states, and it appears to be expanding its territory in spite of massive efforts to contain it. It is estimated that about 136 million acres are now infested. One acre of land may contain as many as a hundred of the large, distinctive fire-ant mounds, some of which reach three feet in diameter. It is easy to imagine how difficult it would be to plow, plant, or pasture such an acre. Unfortunately, the fire ant has not confined itself to farmers' fields. It has become a hazard in ball parks, school play yards, parks, and lawns.

The fire ant derives its name from its sting, which literally burns like fire. The venom differs from that of its Hymenoptera cousins the bee, wasp, hornet, and yellow jacket. It contains a toxic substance that destroys (necrotizes) tissue in the area of the sting. Large, unsightly scars may result. Worse still, there are some people so sensitive to fire-ant venom that a single sting can be fatal. Unlike the bee, the fire ant can sting repeatedly. His lancets are not barbed and can be withdrawn. The fire ant actually bites its victim first. Then, hanging on like a bulldog, it swivels, stinging over and over again. Thus several stings are inflicted within a very small area.

To make matters worse, fire ants can literally explode from their mounds when disturbed. Within seconds, any animal or human being who blunders into their colony is aswarm with hundreds, even thousands, of ants. Pigs, calves, and even horses have been reported stung to death in this manner. A few human fatalities are also on record, although probably the majority of the deaths were due to an allergic reaction rather than a toxic one. No wonder people who live in fire-ant country are deeply concerned about these pests, especially those who live where small children and fire ants can collide. Unfortunately, fire ants also often invade the home as they search for food.

The sting of a fire ant causes a characteristic lesion that differs markedly from the wound of other members of Hymenoptera. A wheal forms and begins to expand at the site, and within four hours small blisterlike sacs (pustules) filled with a thin, clear fluid surround the sting site. As the fluid leaks, or the pustules are ruptured, the centers of the vesicles become depressed. Within eight to ten hours cloudy fluid, which rapidly becomes purulent, appears at the sting lesion. After about twenty-four hours the pus-laden lesion is sometimes surrounded by a thin, red halo or by a much-larger painful, red, swollen area. The lesions remain for three to eight days until the pus is absorbed. Crusts then form, and scar tissue slowly develops. The whole business can be temporarily unsightly, and like other insect stings it can itch like the dickens.

The venom of the fire ant is potent and a very real hazard to those allergic to it. This is what can happen to such a sensitive individual, as recounted by the patient herself:

> I took a break from furniture refinishing and walked back to a little dock at the end of a short causeway extending into the marsh. In turning to leave I stepped on one or two small fire-ant hills, and ants began stinging me around the perimeter of the sneaker on my left foot. Three, possibly four, ants were stinging before I was able to shake off the remainder of the attackers. Having been stung several times before, I noted the usual red blotches about the size of a half dollar which occurred almost immediately, and forgot about them.
>
> About fifteen minutes later my face began to burn, and immediately afterward an increase in my heart rate occurred. Assuming that it was a passing thing, I continued my work for perhaps a minute before deciding that I should alert someone. By the time I got into the house and picked up the phone, my pulse rate was faster than I was able to count, and my face was aflame. After contacting a secretary at the hospital I sat quietly for some five minutes, but when I began having deep pains in the middle of my chest, which I judged to be heart pains, I lay down. The pains soon ceased. Several minutes went by with very rapid heart rate, blurred vision, and general irritability and fear. My face was swollen about the eyes, my eyeballs bright red, and when I attempted to walk about, I felt faint and was forced to again lie down. There was no other pain except the chest pain which lasted perhaps two to three minutes. I had no breathing difficulty[1]

That is a patient's own view of a severe systemic reaction.

A colleague supplied me with the following case of a believer who practiced what his physician preached, an obedience that saved his life. This man had suffered allergic reactions to bee and wasp stings in the past, but had never had any difficulty with ant stings until he went hunting in

[1]Laurie L. Brown, M.D., "Fire Ant Allergy," *Southern Medical Journal* 65:273 (March 1972).

ANTS

Alabama and stepped into a fire-ant mound. Within five minutes he was suffering systemic symptoms of nausea, vomiting, widespread flushing, and asthma. He then lost consciousness. Being a believer, he had along with him the insect-sting kit prescribed by his doctor for his allergy to bees and wasps. A friend who was hunting with him quickly administed the epinephrine contained in the preloaded syringe in the kit. As soon as the victim had recovered sufficiently he was taken to a hospital. He had been stung about fifteen times on the leg, but because he was a believer, he was alive, not dead.

A survey made by Dr. R. Faser Triplett of Jackson, Mississippi, gives an idea of the damage the fire ant can inflict on human beings. Of the physicians practicing in Mississippi, Alabama, and Georgia whom he polled, 901 reported that during a seven-month period in 1971 they had treated 12,438 victims of fire-ant stings. Half of the patients required treatment for secondary infection, 8 required skin grafts, and 5 suffered amputation of a limb. Almost half of the patients exhibited localized allergic swelling, and almost 2,000 exhibited symptoms of a generalized systemic reaction. Of the latter group 76 suffered some form of anaphylactic shock.

These are ants to be avoided.

READER'S GUIDE TO ANTS

Know the enemy:

The harvester ant:
Black or red in color, the harvester is long-legged and often as large as ⅓ inch. **(See Plate 10.)** Its nests are usually large, low mounds bare of vegetation.

The imported fire ant:
Usually red in color, the ants appear to take on the coloration of the soil of their habitat—dark soil, dark ants; black soil, black ants. **(See Plate 11.)** The nests

are mounds of various heights, depending upon the surroundings. Nests on mowed lawns or pastures may be almost flat, and nests elsewhere may be fairly high. (The domestic fire ant also can cause problems, but they are not as prolific or as widespread.)

What to do if stung:

Home treatments:
There is not much in the way of helpful medication for normal reactions to imported fire-ant stings. Minimize the chance of possible secondary infections, such as impetigo, by keeping the area clean and by not scratching during the itching stage. Children's fingernails should be kept short.

Emergency treatment for allergic reactions:
Use the insect-sting kit as directed if one is available, and rush the victim to the nearest physician or hospital. If no kit is available, take the victim to the nearest physician or hospital immediately. An allergic reaction to ant venom—like an allergic reaction to the venom of other Hymenoptera—can progress rapidly from mild to severe, even to fatal, in a matter of minutes

What to expect in long-term management of allergy to ants:

- Immediate initiation of the hyposensitization procedure.
- Prescription for an insect-sting kit with careful instructions in its use and with the suggestion that you keep one on hand at work, at home, and at your places of recreation.
- Suggestion that a warning tag or bracelet be worn to signal allergy to insects.

How to avoid being stung:

- Avoid anthills and mounds.
- Keep legs and arms and feet covered since they are the areas most frequently stung.
- Do not leave food uncovered or uncontained within the house, since this is an open invitation to ants, even fire ants, which do not usually invade the house.
- Treat ant colonies with insecticides recommended by your country agent or the United States Department of Agriculture. The insecticides on the market change from year to year as insecticides that prove too hazardous are removed and new, more effective ones are introduced.

8

Mosquitoes:
The Lady Is the Villain

There are two members of the order of Diptera—which is 85,000 species strong—that we can be certain that we could do without: flies and mosquitoes. Most of us can say nothing good about either of them. But since neither species shows any sign of going into a decline, I suppose that we must learn to cope with their annoyances and depredations. We really cannot get away from them, for they are everywhere—on every continent and in just about every area of every continent, in the city as well as in the wild. There is even one species of fly, called the petroleum fly, that passes through its larval stage in crude oil.

What distinguishes the Diptera from other insects is the possession of only one pair of wings that actually function as wings. They also possess a second, underdeveloped pair that act as stabilizers, particularly when they are flying. Of most concern to us is the engineering of their mouthparts, since this is the instrument with which we become most familiar in our dealings with them. In some of the clan the mouthparts have developed into a long, slender tube, called a proboscis, which is a superior sucking implement to draw off our blood. In other families of Diptera the proboscis is short but functional; in still others the mouthparts are nonessential since the insect lives on the fat it stores up during the larval stage and does not eat at all as an adult.

As an order, the Diptera range from the villainous to the virtuous. Many members are bloodsuckers. Some in the larval stage are scavengers and parasites on animals and other insects. Some bore into plant stems or work over their leaves, while others live in plant galls. Some are predators of many insects harmful to man, and some are pollinators of flowers. A good many are just plain pests as far as we humans are concerned.

The Diptera larvae are legless and for the most part headless, or all but headless. In only a few Diptera families do the larvae possess recognizable heads; most are not much more than a mouth at the front end, without eyes or even jaws. They subsist by shredding food and digesting it outside their bodies with salivary substances, then sucking in the mash that they have made. As pupae some of them are strangely equipped by nature. For instance, some of the fly families possess a little balloon or bladder in their heads. When it is time to emerge, they thrust it out to break the seal of their cocoon. Once free, they retract their balloon and, I suppose, never use it again.

Normally we do not think of the flies and the mosquitoes as cousins. Few of us stop to check on the distinguishing features of the order as we angrily slap at a whining member of the Anophelinae, one of the three subfamilies into which the several thousand species of mosquitoes are divided. Nor do we stop to reckon that the fragile insect that bit us was a female of the species. It is only the female mosquito that is out for blood. She must dine on it in order to be able to lay fertile eggs. The male, under no such necessity, subsists on nectar and plant juices and, as far as we are concerned, lives an inconspicuous and innocuous life. I should add that there are some mosquito species that do not bite at all—it never does to make blanket condemnations.

The female of the species has altered human history now and again. She is the one who spread the yellow fever, for instance, which discouraged Ferdinand de Lesseps and his European consortium so that they allowed Americans to take over the building of the Panama Canal. She is to blame for the spread of such grim diseases as malaria, dengue fever, and equine encephalitis. She does all this damage when she sucks the infected blood of one individual and then goes on to probe for blood on another, providing easy access for the germs that she carries with her. This proclivity for transmitting germs has given her the dubious honor of being one of the world's most prominent disease vectors. Her nuisance factor is strictly secondary.

While mosquitoes come in various colors and sizes, they possess similar features: a round head with two compound eyes, which is fronted by antennae. If one is quick to note such things, one can see that the antennae of the male are bushy in comparison to the slender, threadlike antennae of the female. All mosquitoes have feelers, called palpi, which they operate much as we physicians use our fingers to palpitate the skin of our patients in our search for evidence of disease within the body. The female is well equipped to obtain her meal of blood. She possesses a piercing organ encased in a flexible sheath and two pairs of cutting organs, which, when they come together, form the convenient tubelike proboscis to draw up blood and tissue fluids. With a tiny separate duct she injects salivary secretions into the victim's skin. The salivary secretions dilute the blood so that she can suck it up more easily. Anyone who has ever worked on a thick milkshake with a straw can readily understand the frustrations of trying to suck a too-thick liquid through a tubelike apparatus.

The male adult mosquito does not possess such ferocious equipment. His only function is to mate with the female, then die. A short life but, presumably, a happy one.

The mosquito, like many other insects, passes from egg to larva to pupa to adult. Its metamorphosis is complete. Teachers have found the mosquito life cycle so fascinating that few schoolchildren escape the classroom without learning about the facts of mosquito life. They learn that some mosquitoes lay their eggs on the surface of still, or stagnant, water in "rafts"; that the eggs adhere to each other with a sticky secretion; and that other kinds of mosquitoes prefer to dance just above the water and drop their eggs one by one.

Different species have distinctly different preferences about where they deposit their eggs, but in general they choose ponds, marshes, rain barrels, old tires, puddles, wet surfaces, and the like. There are some interesting variations on this theme. For instance, in Alaska the eggs are laid one summer but do not hatch until the ice and snow melt the following spring. These are the mosquitoes that make life miserable for the caribou on their tundra migrations and for the workers on the pipeline from the North Slope to Valdez in southern mainland Alaska. The floodwater mosquitoes lay their eggs along the banks of rivers and in drying pools that will soon be flooded again. The eggs, or most of them at least, will hatch when the river overflows its banks or the pools refill. Another type of mosquito prefers the rot holes in trees where water collects. Ironically, it was discovered during the New Orleans yellow-fever epidemic many years ago that the mosquitoes were breeding in the funeral urns of their victims. Fortunately, schoolchildren are also taught that, in order to cut down the mosquito population, we must first destroy their preferred breeding places, and youngsters all over America learn to drain puddles, pick up old tires and tin cans, and generally get rid of possible egg-laying sites. Knowing the life cycle and the behavior of insects can pay dividends.

Once laid, the eggs generally sink to the bottom of the puddle in which they find themselves. There they lie dormant for days, or months, until the proper hatching temperature arrives. In warm weather the eggs usually hatch within two to three days. Then the air-breathing larvae rise to the surface to attach themselves, some upside down, some horizontally, using breathing tubes in their posteriors. At this stage, as any schoolchild also can tell you, you can kill them by spreading a little oil over their watery home. They feed on microorganisms in the water, using two tufts of hair to stir the currents and bring the tiny plant and animal creatures to their mouths. They get their name, "wrigglers," from their constant squirming about as they both feed and breathe. They are especially vulnerable and mighty attractive to fish at this stage, and mother mosquito somehow usually has the fore-sight not to deposit her eggs in fish-filled ponds.

After four stages of molting the larvae become pupae, which takes about a week during the summertime. The pupae do not eat, but they stay active, moving about the water with a tumbling action, whence the name "tumbler." Usually after two to three days the adult mosquito emerges from the split-ting pupal shell. As soon as its exoskeleton dries out and har-dens, it is ready to fly. The male will mate and die (his adult life span is rarely as long as a week). The female will bite some warm-blooded creature and lay more eggs. Oddly enough, mosquitoes seem always to pick warm, sunny days to emerge from the pupal shell, as though they instinctively are aware of how helpless they would be without the sun and heat to dry them.

As a rule, mosquitoes stick pretty close to their watery home, but some have been known to migrate forty or fifty miles away from their birthplace. This is especially true of salt-marsh mosquitoes. It is most frequently the females who are endowed with wanderlust; the males stick pretty close to their point of origin. Unfortunately, we have unwittingly car-ried mosquitoes into new areas, especially through interna-tional air travel.

Barring accidents, pesticides, and predators, the adult fe-male mosquito can live as long as three months. Some species manage to hibernate over the winter; their last meal of the season is transformed into hibernation supplies instead of eggs. Still, life for a mosquito is hazardous at best. It is likely that most of them last only a few days or a week or two. Within that short life span the female can guarantee the world a fine crop of young to pester the picnicker and the sleeper for many a hot summer day and night. It has been estimated that in an area highly infested by mosquitoes a single human being could be attacked about six hundred times within an hour. Oddly enough, some mosquito species prefer attacking human beings in the sanctity of their homes, while others are outdoor attackers and rarely invade human premises. Most mosquito species like to make their forays at dawn and dusk, but some will attack at any time during the day (the salt-marsh mosquito displays such an insatiable blood thirst).

In the mosquito-bites-human syndrome the mosquito has definite preferences. Not just any old blood meal will do. The mosquito is fastidious in her fashion. She is clearly attracted to some human beings, and she will pass up others, even if they are side by side. It has been observed, for instance, that when a mother and baby are exposed to mosquitoes the mother will suffer about twenty to thirty bites to the baby's one. In a study in which a hardy family sat out a mosquito barrage, the baby received no bites, the father had three times as many bites as his oldest son, four times as many as his wife, ten times as many as each of his other children. This intrepid father certainly sacrificed himself for science.

Why mosquitoes will bite you and not me has long fascinated scientists. What do you have to attract them that I have not got, or vice versa? Some of the research on this problem demonstrates that the lipids (fats or fatlike substances insoluble in water) on some individuals' skin act as repellents. Perspiration acts as a come-on, inviting hungry mosquitoes to dine, as do carbon dioxide, moist air, and dark colors. In one study using the mosquitoes that carry yellow fever a warm target enticed seven mosquitoes, a wet one 22, and one both warm and wet 358. Warm, wet humans set up reasonably strong convection currents, a kind of aura around their bodies. It is postulated that the mosquito zeroes in on those currents on its random flights. The carbon dioxide emitted in our breath triggers sensors that are located on the female mosquito's antennae and apparently excites her to random flight to seek the source. Why she is attracted to dark colors—black, dark blues, and reds—and somewhat put off by light colors—white, light greens, and yellow—is still a mystery. Scientists do know that some estrogens enhance the allure of moisture, warmth, and carbon dioxide so that women are often the targets of mosquitoes during certain phases of their menstrual cycle, while they may be passed up the rest of the time. Oddly enough, mosquitoes seem to prefer to dine on healthy human beings rather than the ailing. Perhaps the blood is richer.

Thus, if you were to draw up a composite of the person whom the mosquito finds most attractive, it would be a woman with dark, warm skin, perspiring a little and breathing heavily (perhaps just off the tennis court), wearing perfume, healthy as a horse, wearing a navy-blue outfit, taking estrogen, and menstruating. In addition, she would be a restless soul, since moving about is more likely to attract mosquitoes than sitting still. But being attractive to mosquitoes is a dubious honor at best and one that most of us would just as soon forgo. As one of Mark Twain's characters, who had been tarred and feathered and run out of town on a rail, said, "If it wasn't for the honor, I would just as soon have forgone the occasion."

I recently saw a patient who had turned the tables on mosquitoes. When she was ten years old, she suffered a bout of malaria. As a result, any mosquito that bites her dies within five minutes. Better still, she suffers no red wheal or itching at the bite site. She is her own best repellent.

Once a person has been bitten, what brings on the red wheal and that uncomfortable and irresistible itching? It seems strange that anything as small and frail as a mosquito can cause so much discomfort. In the past it was speculated that the wheal and the itch were responses to the mechanical irritation of the biting, or cutting, mechanism of the mosquito's mouthparts or that a toxin was secreted with the bite or even that the mosquito injected histamine. We know now that all those things contribute to the victim's discomfort but that the main culprits reside in the mosquito's salivary secretions. The secretions contain allergenic substances that cause an immediate and a delayed reaction: The immediate reaction of the wheal, the reddish area, and the itching that follow the bite within a few minutes—which are usually gone almost as swiftly as they appear—and a delayed reaction of the pimplelike lesion, which is usually accompanied by some swelling and always by intense itching,—which appears a few hours after the bite. The delayed reaction may last for several hours. The role of the salivary secretions in these reactions was demonstrated when the salivary ducts of mosquito were severed, and her bite then failed to produce a wheal or itch in individuals who had suffered those reactions to prior mosquito bites. As we have noted, the mosquito injects saliva when she bites in order to dilute the victim's blood, the better to suck it up in her proboscis.

A controlled experiment was set up employing the yellow-fever mosquito and British subjects who had never before been exposed to its bites and so were not sensitized to the allergenic substances in its saliva. The experiment demonstrated that human beings go through five distinct stages in reaction to the mosquito's bloodletting. In the first stage there was only a small red mark at the bite site. In the second stage, perhaps a day later, a delayed reaction of wheal and itching occurred. After being dined upon, off and on, for about a month the experimental subjects moved into a third stage: an immediate reaction of wheal and reddened area occurred, and also symptoms a few hours later of a delayed reaction that included that troublesome itch. After further exposure to hungry mosquitoes the subjects continued to suffer the immediate reaction, but the delayed reaction decreased and finally disappeared altogether. The experimental subjects never went beyond stage four, but abundant observation has shown that individuals exposed repeatedly to mosquito bites move into a fifth stage free of either an immediate or a delayed reaction. After a good deal of annoyance they arrive at a stage in which they enjoy a certain immunity. It is a rocky road to such carefree unconcern, however, and not one that the severely allergic can travel with comfort. The mosquito's allergenic potential is not as severe as that of the Hymenoptera, but its salivary secretions can cause severe local reactions on occasion among hypersensitive individuals. The following case is one of many that I have collected over the past few years in a survey of reactions to biting and stinging insects:

> J, a child of three and a half, was bitten by a mosquito on the left cheek while playing in the backyard of his home. When he came into the house, his mother was horrified to discover that the left side of his face was swelling "at an alarming rate." She rushed him off to the family doctor, who treated young J for a severe local reaction. Even so, the boy's face continued swelling "until his left eye and eyebrow were completely out of sight." The swelling began to diminish the following day, but, according to his mother, it took J's face six days to regain its normal size.

A doctor wrote me from Australia that immigrants down under have a great deal of trouble with the mosquitoes there until they have been in residence for a year or two. Then, with some exceptions, their allergic reactions to mosquito bites suddenly vanish. One of the exceptions, a woman the docter treated, could raise a nine-by-twelve-inch bump in response to a mosquito bite. It does seem incredible that so small a beast could make such a mess of the human hide. It is interesting to note that those who suffer the severest reactions often are allergic to something else in the environment or have a family history of allergy.

While generalized systemic reactions are rare in response to mosquito bites, they have occurred. As with any other anaphylactic response, they represent a medical emergency. Other severe reactions are also possible. For example, during a mosquito epidemic in Pennsylvania in 1952, one three-year-old child, who had been exposed to mosquito bites for some time, developed a strange reaction to some bites on her legs and hands. Not only did her hands and feet become swollen but also black-and-blue areas surrounded the bites and extended to even the lower part of her trunk. She then developed nausea, severe vomiting, and fever. Walking became painful as red blisters appeared at the black-and-blue areas. The youngster was hospitalized with a diagnosis of "anaphylactoid purpura" (hemorrhage into the skin, mucous membranes, internal organs, and other tissues). I am happy to relate that the child recovered within a week or so.

The mosquito's greatest threat to man is as a disease vector. As I mentioned earlier, the two diseases that are immediately associated with the mosquito are malaria and yellow fever. Malaria, characterized by chills, fever, and heavy sweating, is caused by a protozoan parasite injected by the mosquito when she bites. It is not an important medical problem in the United States, where about 450 persons contracted it in 1975, but it affects millions of people elsewhere around the world. Once thought under control, it is now on the upswing. Because the price of pesticides has risen sharply with the cost of petroleum products, and because mosquitoes are becoming resistant, the World Health Organization is urging malaria-stricken nations to return to the old control methods of draining swamps and screening homes. Scientists are working hard to develop a vaccine, which is apparently the only bright hope on the horizon. Until then, as recorded long ago by a poet of India of the fourth-century A.D.:

> The green and stagnant waters lick his feet
> And from their filmy, iridescent scum
> Clouds of mosquitoes, gauzy in the heat,
> Rise with his gifts: Death and Delirium.

Yellow fever also is not a medical problem in the United States at the present time, but epidemics are a distinct possibility in other parts of the world (and therefore in our part of it). Reservoirs of yellow-fever-laden monkeys inhabit the jungles, and mosquitoes abound waiting to carry the virus from monkey blood to man. Fortunately, we have a preventive vaccine.

Mosquito-borne encephalitis is closer to home and a distinct threat to our health. A recent outbreak in our country brought almost a hundred deaths and thousands of cases in its wake. There are several forms of this viral disease. The Eastern, Western, and St. Louis strains are the most common in our area of the world. One species of mosquito may be a vector for one form and another species for another form. Horses and birds are the principal reservoirs of the disease in the United States. Encephalitis not only kills but also leaves about 10 percent of those victims who do recover with permanent brain damage or paralysis.

We mentally connect dengue fever with tropical jungles, but this disease, also known as breakbone fever or dandy fever, was once epidemic in Texas. Characterized by pains in the arms, legs, and joints, backache, fever, and an intense headache, it too is caused by virus transmitted by the mosquito from individuals infected by the disease.

We also think of elephantiasis as being a disease of Africa and other faraway places, but Charlestown, South Carolina, once had an outbreak of this weird disease. The southern house mosquito is a carrier of the nematode larval worms that cause it. The larvae of the filarial worm settle in the human lymph nodes, where they mature and multiply. Elephantiasis victims exhibit grossly swollen legs and genital organs. Heartworm in dogs is another filarial worm transmitted by mosquitoes. The adult heartworms can so choke the heart or pulmonary artery by their tangled numbers that death results. They are also occasionally found in cats and in wild carnivores.

We are not yet done with mosquito misdeeds. They occasionally transmit tularemia from rabbits and rodents to man. This disease is characterized by chills, headache, aching pains, fever, and vomiting. It is exceedingly debilitating and sometimes fatal. Mosquitoes also transmit anthrax, which used to be exceedingly fatal but is not less so, thanks to penicillin.

As we can readily see, mosquitoes are more than just pests.

READER'S GUIDE TO MOSQUITOES:

Know the enemy:

Mosquitoes come in various sizes and colors, but all have round heads, a slender proboscis, antennae, and palpi (feelers). They are small and fragile with slender legs. **(See Plate 12.)**

What to do if bitten:

Home treatment:

- Wash the bite area with soap and water. Secondary infection from bacteria transmitted both by the mosquito and by scratching is a possibility. An antihistamine, such as Temaril, and calamine lotion help to relieve itching. If there is much swelling, ice packs should be applied, or ice-cold wet dressings of Epsom salts (one tablespoon of Epsom Salts dissolved in a quart of water; the solution should be dissolved hot, then chilled). Bites that cause swelling in the area of the eyes can be treated with cold compresses of bicarbonate of soda (one teaspoon of bicarbonate of soda to a glass of water). The compresses should be left on the swollen area for fifteen or twenty minutes and then replaced if necessary.

- Be alert for signs of secondary infection, such as impetigo, and if such signs occur, consult your doctor. Emergency treatment for an allergic reaction: Remember that occasionally an individual reacts to mosquito bites with symptoms of a generalized systemic reaction—nausea, dizziness, widespread hives, severe swelling, headache, hemorrhagic skin areas, and lethargy. One patient was reported as drowsy and irritable for three days following mosquito bites. When there are generalized systemic-reaction symptoms, the patient should be taken immediately to the nearest physician or hospital. Such a reaction is a medical emergency. It can be fatal because symptoms can progress swiftly toward anaphylactic shock. See the list of allergic-reaction symptoms in **Appendix A.**

100

What to expect in long-term management of allergy to mosquito bites:

- Desensitization to mosquito bites has been fairly successful for the allergic, although less so than for Hymenoptera-sting allergy. For the individual who suffers a severe systemic reaction to mosquito bites, it is well worth a try.

- There is some possibility that thiamine chloride taken orally may act as a repellent to mosquitoes (and to other insects) when it is excreted through human skin. For some poeple it has its own possible side effects of itching, hives, and a rash.

How to keep from being bitten:

- The use of repellents when outdoors is the best bet. The efficacy of different repellents varies from one individual to the next, and some people may be as sensitive to the chemicals in the repellents as they are to mosquito bites. Since mosquitoes will assuredly discover even the smallest untreated area, and since a determined mosquito can bite through many materials, repellents must be generously applied over all exposed areas of the skin and even to clothing. Do not apply repellents too liberally around or above the eyes; for frequently they can sting badly if perspiration carries the chemicals into the eye itself.

  Despite their name, repellents do not actually repel the mosquito as much as confuse her radar. She is guided to the victim by her sensory organs, which confirm the presence of moisture, warmth, and carbon dioxide. Repellent molecules work by blocking the pores of the sensory hairs on her very sensitive antennae, turning her away from you just in the nick of time.

  Repellents that contain Deet (diethyltoluamide) are

101

probably the most effective. Cut 50 percent with alcohol, Deet has little or none of the greasy feeling that is a drawback of repellents to many people. New repellents found in animals are under study at present in an attempt to avoid the use of some of our more harmful man-made chemicals. The defense repellent that the millipede uses against its enemies, for instance, has been found to work effectively against that horror of the home the cockroach, as well as against ants and flies. Such natural substances hold great promise for a pest-free future in the great outdoors. In the meantime, use a good repellent, wear light-colored clothing, and wear long pants and sleeves in order to expose as little of yourself as possible to the bloodthirsty mosquito.

- To keep the home environment free of mosquitoes, good screening is essential. When camping, screened tents and head nets accomplish a good deal. Preventing the mosquito from existing in the first place is the best of all remedies. It is not a difficult chore to eliminate mosquito breeding places or to turn them into death traps. Anywhere water collects and stands should receive such attention: rain barrels, old tin cans and tires; stagnant puddles, ponds and ditches, hollow stumps and trees, marshy ground—all should be either eliminated, treated with a bit of oil, or drained. Stump hollows and the like can be filled with concrete, and ponds stocked with fish, which delight in dining on mosquito larvae.

  In the past DDT was liberally dispersed over large and small areas to control mosquito populations, but with our recent awareness of the impact on the chain of life of such insecticides, we have foresworn such broadcast methods as much as we can. New ideas of insect control are beginning to appear. For example, one company is working on growth regulators, compounds much like the insect's own hormones that upset its metamorphosis at one stage or another. One such compound is a juvenile hormone which regulates the larval period and its various molts but which must not be present when the mosquito is ready to emerge as an adult. It has been tested and will presumably be widely marketed. Field tests demonstrated that, when this hormone is sprayed over mosquito breeding areas, the mosquito young never emerge from the pupa stage. Biological agents are also being developed for mosquito control. These are diseases that kill the mosquito, usually in its immature stage, but are harmless to humans and most other, if not all other, animals, including insects. Another neat trick is the release of sterile mosquito males to produce instant birth control. The males are irradiated and released in areas where control is sought. This technique reduced and all but eradicated malaria mosquitoes in one five-square-mile area in Central America where it was tested.

In the meantime the average person should use insecticides with care, following directions to the letter. The oils used in such products are often harmful to plants; thus care should be exercised spraying in and about gardens or potted plants. Above all, insecticides should not be sprayed upon the person, for they are not repellents, and their toxic properties can be absorbed through the skin. It does not make good sense to reduce the mosquito population at the expense of the human population. We do not yet fully comprehend the long-range effects of low-level exposure to many of these chemicals, but we do know that some of them are definitely harmful to human health. Keep all such products, including repellents, away from children.

Insecticides and other insect-control measures will be discussed at greater length in a later chapter. **Appendix H** contains emergency measures to take in case toxic materials are ingested, inhaled, or contacted.

9

The Fecund Fly

The curses of mankind have rained down upon the fly from time immemorial, and with good reason. Two—perhaps four—of the ten plagues that swept ancient Egypt have been attributed to this pernicious pest. Disease borne by flies contributed to the downfall of the glory that was Greece, the power that was Rome.

Like their Diptera cousins the mosquitoes, flies come in many sizes, shapes, and colors—variety is the name of the game in the insect world—but all kinds of flies are characterized by the possession of a single pair of membranous wings plus small, knobbed halteres, or stabilizers. All the thousands of different fly species have mouthparts that are adapted for sucking either blood or plant juices. Like mosquitoes they all undergo a complete metamorphosis through a larva and pupa stage. When we leave this general frame of reference, however, we encounter strange variations of appearance and habits.

The habits of some flies are horrendous indeed. There is the screwworm, for example, a fly larva that literally eats its way into the flesh of horses, cattle, and other animals in the Southwest. Wherever the animal is cut or wounded the screwworm fly lays her eggs. When they hatch, usually in less than twenty-four hours, the larvae begin to feed on the animal's flesh within and around the wound. The screwworm fly lives only on the living and the warm-blooded; it does not lay its eggs in or feed on dead or decaying animal matter. Needless to say, it caused tremendous losses for cattle and sheep raisers in the past. The release of sterilized males at last brought these insect Draculas under control.

Another gruesome member of the fly family is the coffin fly, which can penetrate three feet of ground to lay its eggs in decomposing flesh. Then there is the botfly, which lays its eggs on the hairs of a horse's legs, shoulder, or belly. The eggs hatch when the warm tongue of the horse licks at the irritation that they cause to his skin. The larvae then travel to the animal's intestinal tract, where they burrow and dine until it is time for pupation, which occurs when they are voided along with manure. A horse untreated for bot infestation may die from sheer numbers of bot larvae. On rare occasions a bot larva may stray onto a human host, where he will create a creeping myiasis, or burrow, under the skin, which is characterized by intense itching. It is not a serious problem and is easily cured by removing the visible larva.

There are a number of variations on the botfly: the cattle grub, which raises a tumor on the backs of cattle; the sheephead maggot, which deposits living maggots in the noses of sheep and sometimes parasitizes human beings; the head maggot of caribou, elk, and deer—a full roster of unpleasant fly species.

Maggots are a familiar sight in blown meat or decayed animal matter, but it is not quite so well known that, even as late as World War II, maggots often helped soldiers who were wounded and left behind untended for days on overrun battlefields. American field-hospital doctors were somewhat horrified to find the wounds of German prisoners, who were gathered last from the scene of battle, swarming with the ugly white fly larvae, but it was soon discovered that the maggots had cleaned away, or debrided, dead flesh and had left the wound areas almost surgically clean and already beginning the healing process from within. It was a shock to many an assumption of how wounds should be antiseptically treated, but there are probably middle-aged Germans today who owe limbs, if not their lives, to the repulsive maggots.

We should not excuse or honor the fly, but some species are helpful as they prey upon harmful insects. Robber flies are fierce predators. Dance flies kill smaller flies in their strange courtship ritual, during which the male fly presents a dead fly of a smaller species to his intended to keep her occupied during the mating process. This stratagem has undergone some odd variations among different dance flies. In one species the male simply offers the dead fly, while in another he gift wraps it in a web that he constructs with secretions from his front feet. Still another species of dance fly simply hands the female a dummy wrapped in a good bit of webbing. By the time she discovers that she has been fooled, it is too late. Other predator-fly species lay their eggs in the bodies of insects injurious to agriculture. When the eggs hatch, the larvae dine on the bodies of their hosts. One such fly, which is native to Japan and Europe, has been introduced in the United States in an attempt to control the gypsy moth.

The housefly, of course, is familiar to us all (**see Plate 13**). We learn during our school days that it can walk on the ceiling because it has sticky feet and that those same sticky feet bring filth and germs into our homes, onto food and everything else that the fly chooses to stroll on. We are also very much aware of the housefly's nimbleness and alertness, although few people know that it can fly five miles an hour, which is not bad when one considers its size. The much larger horsefly can do thirty miles an hour; its wings are correspondingly more powerful. One patient and methodical researcher found, after examining 380,000 houseflies, that the average fly carries 3,683,000 bacteria about with it. Thus the housefly is a carrier of disease. Because it does not bite, it poses no special threat to the allergic. It simply walks upon filth, then does its best to wipe its feet on our food.

Unfortunately, the housefly is fecund. It has been estimated that a pair of flies mating in April could produce enough progeny by August to cover the earth with forty-seven feet of flies. We are fortunate that nature has devised ways other than our own of doing away with a good many housefly descendants. Yet for the sake of human health too many still survive.

The fly not only walks on filth but also dines on it. It is thus that its feet and the hairs of its proboscis become loaded with bacteria. Flies may also vomit and excrete upon human skin and in human food, both of which contaminate. The housefly has been indicated as the transmitter of typhoid, cholera, salmonella enteritis, bacillary dysentery, shigellosis (a sometimes fatal type of dysentery), and gastrointestinal disease. It does not have to bite to produce human misery.

The housefly has a look-alike that does bite: the stable fly. It is about the same color and size (**see Plate 14**). As its name implies, it hangs out in stables and barns. A bloodsucker, it plagues horses, cattle, and sheep, biting them and then sucking blood with its bayonetlike proboscis. When the weather turns cold, it may seek the warmth of human habitations and will, if hungry, seek a blood meal from human beings.

These look-alikes have different patterns of egg laying. The housefly prefers to lay her eggs in excrement or decaying matter, whereas the stable fly, a bit more fastidious, prefers damp straw or soggy hay. Unfortunately for the livestock, the stable fly is every bit as fecund as the housefly. Her offspring during the summer months reach maturity within two weeks, at which time each new generation is ready to mate and lay between twenty-five and fifty eggs. Small wonder that it takes a computer to estimate the progeny that a single housefly couple could produce by the end of summer.

There are other flies that transmit disease among us. The tsetse fly of Africa carries the protozoa of sleeping sickness among people and a kindred disease among their cattle. In the Near East it has been estimated that almost half the adults are blind in one eye or both thanks to a fly-borne virus transmitted from one infected villager to another. In these same fly-ridden villages a third of the infants die before they are a year old, usually from fly-borne intestinal diseases.

I discussed the sometimes beneficial side of maggot infestation in the wounds of soldiers left behind on battlefields.

Maggot infestation of tissue and organs, called myiasis, is anything but beneficial. Myiasis can occur accidently when an individual swallows fly eggs in food or water. Usually such an infestation is transitory, and the larvae are expelled before they can do any harm. On occasion, a fly that inhabits the eastern part of North America lays its eggs on the skin, and the hatching larvae burrow in to produce boillike lesions. A curious method of introducing eggs into human beings is practiced by the human warble fly. It catches a mosquito, glues a number of eggs to the lower part of the mosquito, and then releases it to go its way. When the mosquito lands on a warm-blooded animal or human being, the eggs hatch suddendly, and the larvae attach themselves to the new host and burrow into the skin. Their wanderings within the body can cause itching, pain, and intense discomfort. There are on record a few cases of myiasis in which eyes were infested and destroyed, and at least one fatality from warble-fly larvae has been recorded. A warble, incidentally, is a tumor that flies of this species produce on the backs of cattle. All in all, myiasis is very unpleasant, and the flies that cause it are worthy of eradication, if only it were possible.

In the United States the flies that most commonly cause allergic reactions among the sensitive are deerflies, blackflies, biting midges, and, less frequently, horseflies. While the last may do the least in damage to human beings, the horsefly is generally far from the least in size. As most of us know it in the United States, it is the giant among the flies. And the fearsome racket it makes matches its physique. Heavy-bodied and none too agile, it lends itself to being swatted. But when it does get in a bite, it can suck a good deal of blood and leave a painful wound. Again, the female is the villain, and the pacific males thrive on plant juices rather than blood. Horseflies can transmit diseases, such as anthrax and tularemia, but they are infamous chiefly because of the ferocity of their bite. They can cause allergic reactions in hypersensitive individuals.

For example, a colleague sent me a case report of a man who was standing in a swimming pool when a horsefly bit him viciously on the head. He made a swipe at the creature and knocked it into the water. He then killed it and identified it as a horsefly. Within five minutes he had developed widespread itching and hives over his body. His face began to swell and then his tongue. He was taken to the emergency room of a nearby hospital, where adrenaline was administered. Both the itching and hives subsided almost at once, although his scalp remained sore, and one side of his face somewhat swollen. He soon recovered completely, but since one never knows where or when one will meet a horsefly, his careful physician supplied him with several disposable syringes filled with premeasured doses of adrenaline, which were to be administered if he was bitten again. The physician also recommended that he begin hyposensitization at once.

In a survey that I made several years ago of insect-bite reactions, physicians reported six patients who suffered systemic symptoms from horsefly bites, such as hives, itching, shortness of breath, nausea and vomiting, and faintness. One young woman went into shock. When horseflies do not confine their attention to horses, they can hurt and harm.

Deerflies are much smaller than their horsey cousins, but they are even more vicious biters and much more persistent in their attempts to draw blood. While they usually attack horses, cattle, deer, and other large warm-blooded animals, they would just as soon dine on human beings. Many a horseback rider has leaned down to squash a deerfly drawing blood from his horse's neck only to have others turn their attention on him. Deerflies can be a nuisance, and their bites painful. Worse still, they rather frequently cause systemic reactions among the sensitive. The following case, which I treated a number of years ago, is a good example of what they can do to the allergic:

In May of 1965, L.B. was mowing the lawn when he banged a pine tree with the mower and apparently disturbed several small insects which he then noticed flying about. They gathered about him and, since he was shirtless, bit him about twenty-two times on his back. He immediately felt as if he were about to pass out but managed to reach his house, where he took three Benadryl [an antihistaminic agent] tablets and held another "white" tablet under his tongue. He did not lose consciousness for a few minutes. He was taken to a hospital, where he was admitted and treated with steroids and Adrenalin. He was discharged three days later. One of the insects involved was obtained for examination and was identified by an entomologist as a deerfly.[1]

Recently a colleague sent me another interesting case of deerfly reaction, this time that of a farmer's wife, who was bitten as she "walked the beans" (hoed thistles from between soybean rows). She was bitten on the toe by a deerfly, and within about fifteen minutes both the toe and foot became greatly swollen. Her face also began to swell. A red rash spread over her body and began itching. She said that she began to feel very faint, and she did lose consciousness. She was taken to a nearby doctor and given "injections" (perhaps adrenaline) and soon recovered. With prior and subsequent deerfly bites she suffered similar symptoms, all of which occurred within fifteen to thirty minutes of the bites. Her last reaction was so severe and threatening that her husband finally "retired her from walking the beans."

There are about twenty-five hundred species of horseflies, deerflies, greenhead flies, and clegs, all of which dwell under the scientific name Tabanidae. The males suck plant juices and may even be helpful in their fashion by preying on soft-bodied insects that harm flowers and crops. But the females are a bloodthirsty lot. Their mouthparts are knife-sharp, the better to cut into their victims. In their search for blood they transmit disease from one animal to another and to human beings. About the only compliment one can pay the females of this fly group is that many of them have pretty eyes—jewel-like, large, and brightly colored.

In general, the bloodthirsty females lay their eggs in batches or layers in foliage overhanging water, on rocks projecting from streams or ponds, and the like. The eggs are often

[1]Claude A. Frazier, M.D., *Insect Allergy* (St. Louis: Warren H. Green, 1969), p. 200.

waterproofed en masse by a special secretion. When they hatch, the larvae fall into the water or mud and then burrow their way to organic matter to feed. Deerfly larvae are equipped practically from the beginning with sharp, biting mouthparts. When the tabanid larvae reach the pupal stage, they move to drier ground, where they emerge two or three weeks later in adult form as the familiar pests.

When we examine blackflies, we may wonder what on earth is the use of these incomparable nuisances. From the human standpoint there seems no reason for their existence, and there are probably any number of species of warm-blooded animals that would agree. In large swarms these small, vicious, hump-backed famale biters have been known to kill chickens, birds, and even small domestic animals. In the Mississippi valley it is reported that they have even killed mules. (**See Plate 18.**)

There are about three hundred different varieties of blackfly, none of them pleasant. Anyone who has fished, camped, hunted, walked, or worked in the great out-of-doors, especially in the northern part of North America from New England across Canada to Alaska, knows that life in the woods would be paradise if the blackfly had never become a part of nature's scheme. Actually, the blackfly persists wherever water runs freely, from the north to the tropics. The female is so eager for blood that she will bite through clothing or find her way beneath it to get at a meal. And there are so many of her like that in some areas they literally drive citizens off the streets and into the safety of their homes. For instance, the citizens of Bullhead City, Arizona, have designated their frantic gestures of flailing at the whining, voracious insects buzzing about their heads as the "Bullhead City Salute." Some residents have even taken to wearing head nets when outdoors to escape the hordes of blackflies that descend on the town from their Colorado River breeding area. The blackflies, also called gnats or buffalo gnats, can clear the golf course, empty the streets, clean the kids out of the playgrounds, and move picnics into dining rooms.

Blackflies lay their eggs in watery places, placing them in

such large quantities on rocks, logs, and water plants that they form a mosslike slime. The larvae glue themselves so tightly to rocks and other underwater resting places that they remain in place even at the lip of a waterfall. They have mouth fans to propel organic matter within reach, but they can also move from one site to another by means of suction cups at their posterior ends. During the pupal stage they spin a cocoon and remain under water. When mature they form a bubble within the cocoon that floats them to the surface, where they pop out as adults ready to fly. The males mate at once; the females, driven like tiny Draculas, begin their search for blood.

The blackfly's bite is painful, and the itching it causes is intense. More than that, it frequently causes considerable local swelling, indicating the presence of a toxic substance. Since the blackfly injects a bit of an anesthetic with her bite, the victim is often not immediately aware that he is under attack. He may be startled to find a trickle of blood on his skin. Soon afterward there may be pain. The itch follows. Generally blackflies go for the lower extremities of their targets, but as the "Bullhead City Salute" attests, this is not an unfailing habit.

Some individuals are highly sensitive to blackfly bites, and they react with generalized systemic symptoms and even with anaphylactic shock. A doctor in Bullhead City stated that, after three or four years of being unmercifully bitten, some residents of the area developed severe allergic reactions. He feared that some would suffer shock symptoms as they became more and more hypersensitive to blackfly toxin. This, of course, could represent a very real threat to life. Some researchers, however, believe that people tend to develop a natural immunity to blackfly bites in the course of time, as they do to the bites of mosquitoes. Others suggest that it is not so much that human beings develop immunity as that blackfly species differ from season to season; some species are more vicious biters with more potent toxins than those of others.

Whatever the case, blackflies can cause alarming reactions, as the following accounts demonstrate. One doctor wrote me about a twenty-eight-year-old woman who suffered anaphylactic shock as a result of blackfly bites. By the time she was taken to medical aid, she had no blood pressure or pulse, but fortunately she responded quickly to epinephrine (adrenaline). In another, less life-threatening situation, a doctor in Minnesota treated a woman whose blackfly bites became as large as two to two-and-a-half inches in diameter and stood out an inch or so from her skin. The wheals, or blebs, were painful when they opened, and they apparently lasted several weeks.

Blackflies, like mosquitoes, have their preferences and will seek their blood meals more often from some people than from others. They will even leave one or two individuals in a group strictly alone to direct their malevolent attentions upon the less fortunate. As far as I can ascertain, no one really knows why, although bright colors and an increase in carbon dioxide appear to entice them. Tobacco smoke, on the other hand, is evidently a repellent; within a group the nonsmoker usually gets the worst of it.

The biting midges are as bad as blackflies. As individuals they are all but invisible, but en masse they can be seen dancing on air over lawns and beaches, especially in spring and fall. Also called no-see-ums or punkies, they come in fifty or more types, most of which prefer to attack other insects, and only a few of which choose the blood of mammals such as ourselves. There is one Oriental biting midge that attacks mosquitoes that have just attacked human beings or other mammals and sucks the blood from the mosquito—a kind of insect hijacking.

Biting midges are generally nocturnal, but they will attack at dawn and dusk and, alas, on dark cloudy days and in the shadows of deep woods. Again the female is the attacker, possessing mouthparts like miniature scissors and a stabbing proboscis, which she plunges into her victim after cutting a small incision in the skin. Midges prefer to live near water, but also thrive where the earth is moist a good part of the time, as it is in the woods where trees shade and cool the ground. Midge larvae call both water and mud home; thus they abound in tidal flats, decaying vegetation, old trees and logs, and the like. Anyone who frequents the shore is well aware that saltwater flats shelter midges by the millions, but they are also numerous in freshwater inlets and around ponds. When the wind blows, midges disperse and disappear, but as the wind dies, they reappear as if by magic, and they are usually on the attack.

While midges can transmit both human and animal diseases on occasion, it is mostly their bite that causes the consternation. Frequently the victim is not even aware of this fragile insect's presence until he has been bitten. The bite itself is initially painful. It can raise welts larger than a mosquito's, and it itches like blazes. It itches so much, in fact, that secondary infection is always a real possibility; only superhuman willpower can keep the victim from scratching hard at the bite site. One type of midge bites so viciously that it not only causes considerable swelling but also may raise a blisterlike vesicle, which soon ruptures to form a weeping sore, which can persist for a number of weeks. More commonly the bites simply hurt and itch and then become welts that are fairly large (especially large in comparison to the insect that does the damage).

Some hypersensitive individuals may react to midge bites with generalized systemic symptoms, such as hives, wheezing, shortness of breath, and a feeling of faintness. For example, a colleague sent me information on a case of a three-year-old child bitten by a "black gnat," in all probability a biting midge. The child's family was on vacation on the Maine coast when the little girl was bitten. Marked local swelling occurred at once, but shortly after the swelling became noticeable, the child began to have breathing difficulties with wheezing and coughing. She was rushed to a hospital emergency room, where she was given adrenaline and antihistamines by injection, and soon recovered. It is remarkable that anything so practically invisible can cause so much mischief.

According to one account Thomas Jefferson suggested that the presence of flies en masse speeded the adoption of the

Declaration of Independence. In that oppressively warm July of 1776 flies from a stable near the meeting room in Philadelphia swarmed to the delegates, biting them repeatedly through their elegant thin-silk stockings. Jefferson is reported to have said, "Treason was preferable to discomfort."

It is wholly understandable.

READER'S GUIDE TO FLIES:

Know the enemy:

- The housefly is short of body, bristly, and somewhat plump, with see-through wings. (**See Plate 13.**)
- The stable fly is about the same size and color as the housefly, but a little larger in the body. (**See Plate 14.**)
- The horsefly is large and heavy-bodied. Some horseflies are all black, and some are black and white. The latter are more of a pest for livestock than for human beings. (**See Plate 15.**)
- The deerfly is smaller than the horsefly. Some are black with yellowish spots on the sides of their abdomens, and some are gray or yellowish-gray with black spots along the sides of their abdomens. (**See Plates 16 and 17.**) The former are almost everywhere. The latter are more common in the western United States.
- The blackfly is small. Its coloring ranges from black to gray. It has short, broad wings and thick legs. Its most distinctive feature is a humpbacked appearance. (**See Plate 18.**)
- The biting midge. These are tiny, almost invisible flies.

What to do if bitten by any of these flies:

Home Treatment:
Begin with a thorough washing of the site with soap and

115

FLIES

water and application of an antiseptic. Flies and filth go together. Thus secondary infection either from contamination by the fly itself or from scratching at the itch is a very real possibility. Signs of such an infection are, as we noted earlier, inflammation, redness, swelling, discharge of fluid, and often some pain. An oral antihistamine is often helpful in relieving itching; an analgesic, such as aspirin, will help relieve pain. Salt or baking soda moistened with water help to relieve pain and inflammation. Wet dressings of Epsom salts also relieve pain and itching. The doctor may prescribe steroid ointments if marked inflammation is present. If secondary infection does occur, he may prescribe oral antibiotics and warm compresses.

Emergency treatment for an allergic reaction:
While generalized systemic reactions to horsefly, deerfly, blackfly, or biting-midge bites are uncommon, they do occur. Symptoms such as widespread hives, nausea, shortness of breath, wheezing, and the like represent a medical emergency. A physician or hospital should be sought at once. See **Appendix A** for symptoms of generalized systemic reaction. Again, I reiterate, *no time should be lost in seeking medical aid.*

What to expect in long-term management of fly bites:
Unfortunately, desensitization to fly bites has not been wholly reliable. However, as with mosquitoes, I recommend that anyone who has had a severe allergic reaction give it a try as a protective measure. Physicians have reported good results in desensitizing to deerfly bites, decreasing severe effects in many cases and even preventing allergic reaction altogether for some individuals.

How to keep from being bitten:
Repellents containing diethyltoluamide, or Deet, are usually effective. Applied properly to the skin of exposed areas and to clothing at points of access, they are ex-

ceedingly helpful. One doctor in Maine recommends that mothers smooth baby oil on their youngsters' skin to "set up a barrier against the black fly's contact with the skin." Thiamine chloride taken orally may also help repel the biting flies, although, as I mentioned at the close of Chapter 8, it may have its own side effects for a few individuals.

The use of repellents, attention to sanitation around the home, good screening, and a careful use of insecticides are about the only means of discouraging the vicious members of Diptera at this time. As with the mosquito, new control methods, including growth regulators and sterilization of males, are being developed.

10

Spiders—the Good and the Bad

Back in the days of mythical antiquity it did not pay to challenge in any form or fashion a god or a goddess. Arachne, a maiden of Lydia, should have known better. But pride goeth before a fall, and she was a bit too proud of her skill at spinning and weaving. She has been spinning and weaving ever since, although in a somewhat different form. The goddess Athene took offense at the superior beauty of Arachne's weaving and destroyed her masterpiece, but when the lovely lady from Lydia tried to hang herself in her despondency, Athene loosened the rope and transformed Arachne into a spider. The rope became the cobweb. So goes the tale, which is the source of the name Arachnida for the class of Arthropoda to which spiders belong.

Although we tend to lump spiders with bugs, beetles, bees, and butterflies, they are not really insects; they do not belong to the class Insecta. They have found their way into this book on the health effects of insects upon human beings only because most of us consider them as insects in common parlance.

It is helpful to know what distinguishes Arachnida from Insecta. Spiders have four pairs of legs to the insects' three and a two-part division of their bodies instead of the insects' three-part division. They do not have antennae, a feature that is always found in Insecta. They always possess spinnerets, the truly marvelous organs that produce the web.

Cobweb is probably one of the strongest substances for its size and thickness to be produced by any living creature, including human beings. The dragline of the spider, the thin strand that it hangs upon and uses as a bridge to run the lines of its web, has a strength equivalent to fine tensile steel, although it may be no more than a millionth of an inch in diameter.

It is unfortunate that spiders have developed such a fearsome reputation. This is so despite Robert Bruce and the busy spider that taught him the lesson of "try, try again." We tend to squash a spider the instant we see one. Housewives as a group are intolerant of webs in dim corners. Yet, of the approximately forty thousand different kinds of spiders that inhabit the earth, only a few are harmful to human beings, and for the most part those would rather not have anything to do with us, given a free choice. Spiders do not seek us out to inflict damage. Many will not even bite when handled. One woman, who has developed an industry from spiders by collecting their web strands for gunsights and the like, claims that even the feared black widow is actually a very gentle creature. She handles them constantly without being bitten. I would not, however, recommend being playful with black widows. Their venom is deadlier than that of the rattlesnake, although fortunately it comes in far smaller quantities. It acts upon the human nervous system much as cobra venom does.

Perhaps what makes spiders so feared and so repulsive to us is their manner of dining upon other Arthropods. Spiders and other members of their order (the Araneida) can take their meals only in liquid form. They digest their victims outside their own bodies, then suck in the resulting mush. They create a liquid diet out of the victim by mushing it up with their mouthparts or by making a wound in its body and pouring digestive enzymes into either the wound or the mush that they have made. They suck the resulting food into their digestive system, and only the dry shell of the prey is left, to be dropped from the web. It is something out of a grade-B TV horror, all right.

Spiders do not suck blood. Neither do they eat insects already dead. They will not even attack a living insect as long as it remains immobile. Their prey must be moving, and this makes for some difficulty in keeping captive spiders nourished. Tiny bits of meat must be hung on a thread and dangled in a somewhat lively fashion to entice the spider to pounce and to eat.

Generally spiders live alone, but there are a few species that live in colonies and employ communal procedures to capture and then share prey. One species so successfully builds a better mousetrap that human inhabitants of their environs bring branches decorated with their webs into their homes to serve as flypaper. Some people also allow spiderwebs within their dwellings to rid the home of flies and other pest insects, just as in some parts of Southeast Asia the little gecko lizards are tolerated, even invited, to pursue flies and roaches up and down the walls.

Most spiders are such solitary creatures that, when it comes time to propagate the next generation, the female may have never seen a male spider before and may attack him, thinking he is either food or the enemy. Sometimes, to overcome such misconceptions or out of respect for her appetite, he brings her a bit of dinner when he comes courting. While it is not at all certain that he will be canibalized after mating, a wise male spider hastily withdraws from the scene, lest his lady's appetite recover too quickly. In any case, the males will die soon after mating. Many females die after laying their eggs, although young females may survive through the winter. Some species, such as the black widow, often live for several years.

As is probably well known to almost everyone, spider webs are traps. They come in various forms, but the main purpose is to entrap insects as they fly or saunter past. The spider sits off to one side and rushes out when prey twitches the web. Commonly the hapless victim is swathed in a cocoon for storage but if hungry the spider begins its horrifying meal immediately. If a dangerous adversary, such as a wasp, is caught in the web, the spider can squirt silk about an inch from its spinnerets to immobilize the enemy without coming close enough to be stung. But spiders do not spin webs just to snare dinner. Webs form the nest that shelters the egg cases and the newly hatched spiderlings. Some species do not build snare webs at all. They have a correspondingly different silk, which lacks the adhesive quality of that used to construct webs to catch and hold prey. While male spiders spin silk, only the female spider possesses the kind of silk that is wrapped around egg cocoons—a marvelous division of assets. The webs of different species often are characteristic—some are sheets, some tubes, some geometrical. The black widow's web is characteristically untidy, for instance. There are cases on record in which fires have been started by spiders that have constructed their webs from the pilot lights of gas stoves to wooden walls or furniture.

When they emerge from the egg cocoon, spiderlings come equipped with built-in larders: their midgut is packed with nutritious yolk, which they slowly absorb. But their digestive systems are incomplete, and they cannot yet manage ingested food. Initially they stay in the web that their dead mother constructed for them or—if she is of one of the more fortunate long-lived species—they ride on her back or remain in a brood cocoon that their mother guards zealously. When the yolk is depleted, the spiderlings' digestive systems have become fully developed, and hunger strikes. They occasionally dine upon each other, but generally a built-in desire to go out and see the world matures along with the digestive tract, and they scatter in all directions before cannibalism really sets in.

For a spider the business of going out into the world can be as simple as running off in any direction. In some species it gets a bit more complicated and a great deal more interesting. The spiderling climbs something—a bush, a branch, a tall weed—as high as it can go and then spins a strand of silk. When a breeze comes along and catches at the thread, the baby spider lets go, and off it sails like an accomplished balloonist. Spiderlings have been observed sailing their threads five miles above the earth and hundreds of miles out to sea. When they finally do come in for a landing, their adult life begins. They build their web or burrow or just wander about under rocks and leaves as their instinct dictates.

All spiders possess venom. The quantity and toxicity varies from species to species. Only a very few species can inflict damage upon human beings. Several spiders within the United States can do considerable damage with their bite: the black widow, the brown recluse, and, far less than its reputation, the tarantula, as we shall see in the next chapter.

The black widow probably heads the list of toxic species. The female is distinctive and would stand out in any spider crowd if spiders were sociable. Usually shiny black—there is also a brown-widow spider—she has an hourglass marking on the underside of her abdomen, which may be bright red, orange, or sometimes, yellow in color. She is the fat lady of the spider world; her gross abdomen often is distended with eggs or food. Her legs, however, are long and slender, the better to scurry away or to grasp her prey. The male black widow—one does not call him a widower—is smaller and not nearly as fat or shiny. Nor does he bear the distinctive hourglass, a marking that is situated in such a way that it is a real trick to identify the black widow in time to avoid it. The widow spiders, black or brown, derive their name from the female's habit of at least occasionally consuming the male after mating, but there is some question about how habitual to the species this unloving performance actually is.

The black widow inhabits the Western Hemisphere from Canada to Chile. It lives in every state of the union. Its relative the brown widow is found mainly in the South. We come upon the widow spiders more often in the late summer and early fall.

The widows are shy by nature and would just as soon have no dealings with us, but when pushed or hurt, they will bite, and they are very poisonous. As I said earlier, the venom of the black widow is more deadly than that of the rattlesnake, measure for measure. In fact, it is fifteen times more potent when it is compared by weight in a dried form. The venom of the brown widow is not nearly as potent. People are bitten more by accident than because of any purposefulness on the part of the black widow, although she will bite to protect her egg cases. Generally she bites when disturbed in hiding places, such as boots or shoes, clothing or bedding, under rocks, in log piles, near her webs in dark corners and under houses, and in baskets or boxes. Once in a while her remains are found in canned goods, part of the seemingly inevitable insect and rodent debris that finds its way into food products. Experiments have demonstrated that her venom has no effect if ingested under such conditions, though the thought is not pleasant.

Variously called the shoe-button spider, the hourglass spider, or the T spider, the black widow constructs its untidy webs in dark places, such as dry crevices in rock walls and rock piles, under trash, in dim corners of barns and outbuildings, in privies (at least in the old days), among logs, and in woodpiles—wherever it can live in peace and return swiftly when danger threatens. The female black widow suspends her large white or tan egg cases in her web, usually during the midsummer months. Each case, or sac, contains around six hundred eggs, which would make a lot of black widows. Fortunately for us, mortality runs high among the newly hatched spiderlings. Unless there is an immediate and ample food supply in their vicinity, they dine upon each other. In fact, mother may join the feast to consume a goodly number of her own young. We may deplore such behavior, but it is just as well that thousands of black widows do not survive in our environs each summer. Some of us, I guess, would even cry, "Go to it!"

After the black widow catches an insect larger than itself in its distinctive, oddly spun web, it rushes out and swathes the struggling victim in a webbing of strong silk, staying at a safe distance as it does so until it has it wound up like mummy. Only then will the spider approach and inject its venom. When the victim dies, it sucks the fluid from the body and, being a good housekeeper, cuts the remains loose from its web to drop to the ground. Thus it disposes of the garbage. Sated, the black widow then waddles back to its hiding place to await the next meal to be entangled in the exceedingly strong strands of its unhandsome web.

The female black widow is not the only poisonous member of her family, although she is by far the most potent. The male's venom is also toxic, and so, oddly enough, are the egg sacs. The latter are so poisonous that care must be taken when destroying them. One study demonstrated that when two egg sacs were crushed and mixed with a drop of saline solution, an injection of the mixture could kill a mouse or even a rabbit.

Although its venom is potent, the bite of the black widow is not invariably fatal. About 5 percent of those who are bitten and untreated die. A number of factors affect the severity of the symptoms that the venom produces. The size and maturity of the spider and the health and the age of the victim make a difference in the potency of the venom and the victim's ability to withstand it. The number of times the victim is bitten and the amount of venom injected naturally affect the outcome. The location of the bite is also a factor.

Frequently the victim does not remember being bitten, although he may recall a pinprick of pain, followed by a dull ache in the region of the bite. It takes a little time for the pain to register, but when it does, it increases in intensity and continues for twelve to forty-eight hours before slowly decreasing. Victims bitten on a finger have described the pain as being like a red-hot poker thrust progressively up the arm. Muscle spasms and rigidity are common symptoms. Typically, the muscles of the abdomen become hard and "boardlike," often with accompanying tenderness. This symptom appears to be especially common if the bite is on the leg. If a hand or arm is bitten, the pain usually occurs in the back, chest, or shoulder and is especially intense when the victim draws a breath. Other possible symptoms include nausea, vomiting, convulsions, paralysis, cold sweats, discoloration of the skin, breathing difficulties, insomnia, delirium, and shock. The most persistent symptom, however, is severe abdominal pain, so severe that the victim draws up his legs against his body. He may groan frequently and be restless and anxious.

In what can be considered a typical encounter with a black widow, a three-year-old girl playing in a garage attached to her home suddenly called out to her mother that there was a bug on her neck. The mother ran out and was horrified to find a black widow in the child's hair and two small puncture wounds on her neck. She rushed the child to the hospital. By the time she was seen by medical personnel, the little girl had started to complain of headache and abdominal pain. Even as the doctor examined her, she groaned and vomited, and the boardlike rigidity of her abdomen became increasingly apparent. The strange part of the case is that she did not complain of any pain in the bite areas, and the bite itself was so small that it could have gone unnoticed. The child was given antivenom and steroids, and an ice pack was maintained on the neck wound. Within six hours after treatment was begun, she began to feel better, and she was discharged from the hospital the next morning. Prompt and proper treatment makes the difference.

If the small puncture wound of the black widow's fangs is missed, there is some danger of misdiagnosis. The symptoms of severe abdominal pain and rigidity mimic the symptoms of several possible illnesses that call for immediate surgery, such as ruptured peptic ulcer, intestinal obstruction, red-hot appendix, and the like. Thus it is vital that the victim and those about him give the physician an accurate account of the progress of the symptoms and of the circumstances under which the victim became ill. For example, a man removing a heap of stones or a pile of accumulated trash who suddenly develops pain and other symptoms described above could easily have encountered a black widow during his work. For instance, when I was a senior medical student, I encountered a man in the emergency room who was scheduled for surgery for a possible ruptured appendix. He looked like a "good ole country boy." I asked an accompanying relative where the patient lived. On a farm? Yes. Got a bathroom? No. Privy? Yes. Had he been to the outhouse? Yes. Felt anything, perhaps a prick of pain? Yes. I looked. Sure enough the marks of the black widow were there.

Cleopatra once clasped an asp to her bosom to speed her way out of this world. It may seem incredible, but, according to one physician, a man attempted suicide by inducing a black widow to bite him. He had been bitten several years earlier by a black widow and treated in time, and he must have gotten the idea from the earlier experience. The unhappy man was successfully treated again.

Until recently, the brown recluse spider was virtually unknown to the general public. It came out of the South and Middle West and was most numerous in Missouri, Oklahoma, and Arkansas. It appears to have migrated as far east as Georgia and as far north as Illinois, and it may turn up as far north as Maine. A colleague sent me a clipping from a Portland, Maine, newspaper about the death of a woman who may have been bitten by a brown recluse. According to the clipping, there had been only one prior sighting of a brown recluse in New England. The brown recluse seems to have arrived in the United States from nowhere, but the symptoms of its bite and its exceedingly toxic venom have been recognized in South America for almost a century. The first case of a brown-recluse bite here was documented in 1957.

Smaller than the black widow, the brown recluse's color ranges from dark brown to tan. Its distinctive mark is a fiddle-shaped band of darker color running back from the area of its eyes to the juncture of the two sections of its body. Its body is about three-eighths inch long, but its legs are long and slender. While it may be found outdoors, it prefers human habitations and outbuildings. Like the black widow it spins irregular webs in dark, out-of-the-way places and in the folds of unused or infrequently used clothing where it is unlikely to be disturbed. Outdoors it is especially fond of rock piles and spaces under leaves. Indoors it favors attics, basements, closets, the undersides of steps, the area around water heaters, and the like. It is very shy and as retiring as its name implies, but unfortunately, since it frequents human habitations, people do get bitten.

The venom of the brown recluse is damaging, to say the least. It can be fatal, but only rarely is so. It is most dangerous to young children, to the elderly, and to those in poor health. In spite of the damage the venom eventually can do, the victim of a brown recluse is often unaware that he has been bitten. The initial symptoms are very mild: perhaps a little stinging sensation but very little pain, if any. Within two to eight hours the bite site does begin to hurt, although the pain varies from not much to a great deal. A slight rash appears in the bite area; then a blister forms. If the victim recognizes the reactions as symptoms of a brown-recluse bite and gets himself quickly to his doctor before other symptoms begin damage from the necrotic mechanism in the venom may be contained, and systemic symptoms may be avoided or lessened in intensity.

Untreated, the lesion appears to harden in the center, as the rash increases in area. In three or four days the center of the lesion turns dark with radiating points. At the end of a week the area looks thoroughly gruesome: the flesh is ulcerated, and the center is depressed and sharply defined. Even so, there often is little pain associated with the horrifying-looking process. Systemic symptoms often develop, and they can be serious, especially in children. Fever and chills, malaise, nausea and vomiting, weakness, and small purplish spots over the skin may appear within twenty-four to forty-eight hours following the bite. Occasionally there is gangrene in the bite area. A life-threatening condition may develop called hemolysis, which is the destruction of the red blood cells. One symptom of it is red-tinged urine.

All this is grim indeed, but the possible effects of the bite of the brown recluse are in dispute at this time. One faction suggests that a great many people are bitten by this spider with no greater consequences than a light rash and some swelling and that more severe reactions are the exception rather than the rule. The male brown recluse is not nearly as potent as the female. Thus those who are bitten by him receive a much less dangerous venom. The brown recluse is fairly abundant in the South and Southwest. Large numbers of them have been found, for instance, among the cliffs in northwest Arkansas. They are often found in grassy and weedy fields in those regions. It seems highly possible that a good many individuals encounter them in and out of their homes and outbuildings and get bitten as a consequence. The more sensational results of the bites may find their way into clinical studies. The perhaps-more-common reactions of rash and swelling and nothing more may not even get to a doctor's office, much less into his notes on clinical observations. Nevertheless, until the controversy is settled, I recommend that a physician be consulted when the initial symptoms of rash, swelling, and some pain and a blister follow a possible brown-recluse bite. Since many victims are bitten while they sleep and find the symptoms only when they awaken, the possibility of a brown-recluse bite may never enter their minds. Even so, remember the brown recluse when such symptoms develop, especially if the victim is a child, an elderly person, or one in poor health. Conceivably, bearing the danger of the brown recluse in mind could save a life.

READER'S GUIDE TO SPIDERS:

Know the enemy:

- The female black-widow spider is black and has a shiny, fat, roundish abdomen and a red or orange hourglass marking on the underside of the abdomen. **(See Plate 19.)**
- The female brown-recluse spider ranges in color from dark brown to tan. A characteristic darker fiddle-shaped mark runs back from the area of her eyes almost to her abdomen. **(See Plate 20.)**

What to do if bitten by a black widow:

Home treatment:

- Seek medical help as quickly as possible.

- Immediate first-aid steps can also be taken. Place ice packs on the bite immediately to slow the absorption of the venom. As with all bites, the wound should be disinfected. Some authorities recommend placing a tourniquet between the bite and the heart; others state that this will only add to the victim's discomfort. If a tourniquet is applied, remember it must be loosened about every five minutes.

- It is helpful to salvage the spider that did the biting since positive identification is always a plus in treating the patient.

Emergency treatment:

Emergency medical treatment of black-widow bites by the physician consists of antivenom. This counteracting serum was first developed by an Argentine doctor, Dr. R. R. L. Sampayo, who used horses to obtain it. He gradually built up the strength of injections of venom into the animals until they developed sufficient tolerance to it. Antivenom has proved a lifesaver, effective even when it has been judged that the victim received a lethal dose. If administered early enough, it will prevent much of the intense agony that generally follows a black-widow bite, and it provides relief from other symptoms quickly, often within an hour or two.

The second aim of treatment is to relieve the intense pain that so frequently develops. Muscle relaxants, hot baths, and calcium-gluconate solution given intravenously are administered to this end.

SPIDERS

What to do if bitten by a brown recluse:

Home treatment:
- Transporting the victim immediately to medical help is the first priority.
- Retrieve the spider so that a positive identification and diagnosis can be made. Because there are a number of brown spiders that bite.
- Apply an antiseptic and ice packs to the bite immediately.
- Do *not* apply a tourniquet.
- Do *not* treat as a snakebite by cutting at fang marks or applying suction.

Emergency medical care:
As yet there is no antivenom for the brown recluse. Physicians have reported good results with the use of steroids and antihistamines and antibiotics. The unsightly lesion that may result from the bite will be slow to heal and sometimes is so extensive as to require grafts.

What to do if bitten by other species of spiders:

- Almost all spiders possess venom of some degree of potency, although the venom of none of the others approaches that of the black widow or the brown recluse in toxicity. Spiders not only possess venom but also are capable of causing allergic reactions, sometimes very severe ones, in the hypersensitive. Thus it is necessary to be alert for signs of a systemic reaction following any spider bite and to get the victim to a doctor at once if such symptoms appear. Allergic reactions may be immediate or delayed; see Appendix A for details.
- All spider bites should be washed and disinfected.

Spiders: The Good and the Bad

How to keep from being bitten by spiders:

- Keep rubbish and dirt where spiders could find a place to hide, from accumulating in outbuildings and in the home area.
- Let light into dark areas as much as possible.
- Always wear gloves when handling old piles of scrap, lumber, rocks, and the like.
- If you suspect a lurking brown recluse within the home, spray baseboards (especially in closets and behind furniture that is not often moved) and behind pictures and the like with a household insecticide.
- Always shake out clothing or bedding that has remained undisturbed for any length of time before using it.
- Do not leave stacks of newspapers, old clothing, and the like undisturbed in attics or basements.
- Sweep or vacuum closets and corners frequently and around water heaters.
- Bring down spiderwebs with a broom.
- Take care in destroying egg sacs. They are best burned quickly.
- Precautionary measures are especially worthwhile in areas where children play, for youngsters are not only the most frequent victims of spider bites, they are also the most vulnerable.

11

Tarantulas and Scorpions

The tarantula is in appearance one of the most awesome of the Arachnids. Large and hairy, with legs several inches long, it has inspired fear and loathing through the ages. Its fearsome reputation, at least in the United States, is generally undeserved. Tarantulas are not very poisonous, and, in fact, they should be considered man's good friends, since they destroy a good many pest insects. They are not aggressive and have to be pushed to bite. They cannot make prodigious leaps of ten to twenty feet as the tales would have us believe. However, because of their fierce looks and their fierce reputation, at least one jeweler in the land has set a tarantula in his display window to guard his treasures while the store was closed at night. It rather teases the imagination to conjure up a would-be jewel thief whose stealthy hand moves among the treasures on display and encounters a six- or seven-inch tarantula. Heart attack? Perhaps.

The tarantula is said to derive its name from the seaport town of Taranto, Italy, whose inhabitants were afflicted with a peculiar disease, a hysterical malady called tarantism. Melancholy characterized by dull, stuporous behavior would give way to a franctic mania for wild, frenzied dancing. Somehow, perhaps from sheer terror, the people of the area would break into the same delirous dance after being bitten by a tarantula. They believed that perspiring profusely would drain off the venom before it could do harm. Taranto and tarantism are apparently the origins of the names *tarantula* for the creature and *tarantella* for the overly exuberant dance.

We call our large spiders tarantulas as people in South America do, but their collection includes some unusual large spiders that we are spared. One is so large that it even captures small birds such as hummingbirds. It usually attacks them while they are hatching their eggs in their nests. As is the wont of the spider family, it sucks the bird dry of its bodily fluids. South American tarantulas can also be very poisonous, and their bite is a great deal more painful than that of our mild and gentle North American species.

Tarantulas do not spin webs. They snare their victims with their many swift feet. They live in burrows in the ground, which they line with their silk. There they stand guard over their cocoons and their young. They are able to survive the winter in their burrows by covering them over with silk and remaining dormant in them until warm weather comes again. Thus they can survive several years.

All in all, the tarantula is much maligned in the United States. Our tarantula species are far less to be feared than the black widow or brown recluse. It is no wonder that some people have begun keeping them as pets (although those who do so should be wary of their tarantulas' origins, lest they acquire one of the very poisonous South American species).

No one in his right mind would keep a scorpion as a pet. Of all the Arachnids in America this is the one that can do the most damage. Its sting can hurt like fury, and it can be fatal, especially for young children.

The scorpion does not resemble its spider cousins in the least. Rather it looks like a miniature lobster or crayfish, for it is equipped with pincers that look for all the world like claws. It holds these out in front and always at the ready as it moves about. With the pincers it can grasp and hold its prey while it brings its potent stinger into action. Its stinger is really its tail, which it carries raised and thrust forward over its back. Poison glands are situated at the end of the tail in a bulbous sac to which the stinger is attached. Unfortunately for the victim, be it insect, animal, or human, the scorpion can sting repeatedly once its stinger has made contact. Anyone who wanted to keep a scorpion as a pet could clip off the stinger segment of its body, and it could keep on functioning quite well, although it would still be far from cuddly.

Gray, brown, yellowish, or black in color, the scorpion comes in various sizes ranging anywhere from one-half inch to eight inches. About 650 species inhabit the earth. About thirty of them are in the United States, mostly in the dry southwestern regions. Of those thirty species only two possess exceedingly toxic venom. They are mainly in southern Arizona, and they can be recognized by their lemon or greenish-yellow color. The size of a scorpion bears no relation to its lethality. The fearsome-looking giant hairy scorpions of the Southwest are timid creatures who can inflict a painful bite but not a potently toxic one, while much smaller scorpions found in that area and in Mexico can kill.

Like most other spiders the scorpion is a loner. When it meets another scorpion, it remains in its vicinity only to mate or to fight to the death. In the latter event the loser often provides dinner for the victor. In mating, if the male does not beat a hasty retreat, his light-o'-love may also dine upon him. No wonder that it pays scorpions to lead a solitary life under stones, in rock crevices, under the bark of trees, or amid piles of trash. During the dry seasons scorpions hide in the ground, but when the rains come, they surface and seek shelter under loose stones. Thus they are more often seen when the weather is wet, which is not too often in the habitat of most species. So many pop up during a rain in the arid and semiarid regions that they inhabit that people might think it had rained scorpions—a horrible thought.

Scorpions frequent outbuildings and homes on occasion. There are cases on record of individuals who were stung by scorpions that found their way into beds. Nocturnal by habit, a scorpion may go unnoticed once it gets into a house. It may arrive, in an attic for instance, by climbing between wall partitions. To be near water, it favors kitchens and bathrooms. It likes to hide in shoes, folded blankets, or heaped clothing during daylight hours and come out after dark to wander. Children's backyard sandboxes are a favorite place for scorpion burrowing.

Like other members of its class the scorpion grows by molting. The old skin is shed along the line of the fore- and the midgut and takes with it the lining of both and the lining of the "book lungs," the breathing organs along its sides. Scorpions are the Methuselahs of the Arachnids: they live three to five years, and they reach maturity very slowly, perhaps because they are able to go for months, even a year, without food or water. When the male reaches maturity, he goes about seeking a mate. When he finally meets his lady, they engage in an elaborate courtship dance. He grasps her pincers, and they rub their lethal tails as they dance. At least by waltzing her around he postpones his demise. The young are born alive, encased in a thin membrane, twenty to forty at a time. Mother helps the baby scorpions get untangled, and they climb on her back, hanging on with their tiny pincers. She flattens herself closer to the ground to make it easier for them to assume the piggyback position. They remain up there, for about a week or so, carried about by their seemingly overloaded mother, subsisting on yolk that is packed in their midguts. Their first molt occurs up there on mother's back. After this the youngsters become more active and begin to drop off one by one to venture out into the world on their own. Now the yolk is gone, the midgut is empty, and presumably the young scorpions are very hungry. They do not, however, feed upon mother, as legend would have us believe. They may on occasion dine upon each other, especially right after that first molt, when their exoskeletons are still soft and their yolk is gone. In fact, mother may dine upon them if they do not scatter with reasonable dispatch. The debris left upon her back after that first molt—all those baby scorpion skins,— gives her a very disheveled appearance. She looks definitely chewed upon.

Odd legends surround scorpions. They supposedly will commit suicide by stinging themselves if surrounded by fire.

It is true that scorpions cannot survive intense heat. When they cannot escape it, they strike about with their tails as if trying to sting. It is the temperature that kills them, however, not their own venom. Some folk tales would have it that scorpions will form a living chain to hang down from ceilings just to sting a passing human. One folk remedy advises the victim of a scorpion's sting to mount an ass and whisper in its ear that he has been stung by a scorpion. The pain is then supposed to be transferred to the poor beast.

Some of the world's scorpions are real killers. In Egypt scorpions bring death to about 60 percent of the children under five who have the misfortune to be stung. One species in Mexico is responsible for many fatalities. Even Europe shelters a species whose venom is potent enough to kill. The European hedgehog is oddly immune to scorpion venom,—and to that of the European poisonous snakes—but dogs and birds will quickly fall victims to it. Modern methods of transportation cause exotic fauna to turn up a good distance from their native habitats. A scorpion traveled with some fruit all the way from Texas to Canada to find a victim.

The venom of American scorpions comes in two potencies. The run-of-the-mill scorpion's sting hurts quite a bit and may cause a local reaction of swelling and perhaps discoloration. On occasion the swelling may be severe, for instance, moving from a stung hand all the way to the armpit, but unless the victim is allergic to the venom, the sting will not result in a serious problem. On the other hand, the venom of the two extremely poisonous species found in the United States mainly affects the nervous system. Little or no swelling or discoloration follows the sting at the wound site. The victim may feel a sharp prick of pain when he is stung, followed by the pins-and-needles feeling that one gets when an arm or a leg goes to sleep. He may then go through a period of hypersensitivity to sensation, but this state soon reverses to one of drowsiness and numbness. His nose, mouth, and throat may begin to itch, his speech may be impaired, and his jaw muscles may contract so forcibly that it is difficult for him to take oral medications. As the nervous system becomes more affected, muscles begin to twitch, and painful muscle spasms occur. The victim may vomit, be incontinent, and go into convulsions. The convulsions may come and go, exhausting the patient, and in this manner may kill him, although it is usually respiratory or circulatory problems that cause scorpion-bite fatalities. Again, it is most frequently the very young and the elderly who die from a scorpion's sting. Children under five are the most susceptible. In a study made in Arizona it was found that scorpions caused about 68 percent of the fatalities from the stings and bites of poisonous creatures. A strange secondary poisoning fatality has even been attributed to a scorpion: scorpion venom in the bloodstream of a woman who had been stung passed into her breast milk to kill her baby.

Down in El Paso, Texas, some mothers go out every morning into the yards where their youngsters play to pour boiling water down scorpion burrows. This may sound like excessive caution, but a survey of Arizona physicians revealed that during a ten-month period they treated 1,573 victims of scorpion stings. Of this number, 233 had to be hospitalized.

To determine whether a small child has been stung by one of the two lethal species of scorpions, doctors in scorpion country tap the sting site gently. If the child cries out in pain or pulls back from the tapping, it almost certainly has been stung by a lethal variety. The stings of the nonlethal species are not particularly painful to the touch at the sting site.

Centipedes, like tarantulas, are somewhat maligned. About 150 different species have been recognized in the United States. Some of them attain a length of six to eight inches. People out West, where those monsters live, naturally fear them. They can bite, and they are venomous, but although their bite can be painful, it is rarely dangerous. Some species invade the human nasal tract and intestinal and urinary tracts (the latter through accidental swallowing). While this is unpleasant to think of, it is also a rare occurrence.

READER'S GUIDE TO TARANTULAS, SCORPIONS, AND CENTIPEDES

Know the enemy:

- The tarantula is large, hairy, and black or brown in color, with legs several inches long. **(See Plate 21.)**
- The scorpion looks like a very small lobster or crayfish. It is gray, black, or yellowish in color and varies in length from ½ inch to 8 inches. The poisonous species have lemon or greenish-yellow coloring in the tail area where the stinger is located. **(See Plate 22.)**
- The centipede has a distinct head and a segmented body, of which each segment has a pair of legs. Color varies. **(See Plate 23.)**

What to do if bitten by a tarantula:

- Do not panic. Tarantulas are not particularly poisonous.
- Wash the bite area well with soap and water to disinfect (one experimenter who allowed himself to be bitten found that hot water on the wound area relieved the pain).
- Consult a doctor if any systemic (allergic) symptoms develop. **(See Appendix A.)**

What to do if stung by a scorpion:

Home treatment:

- Place a tourniquet between the sting site and the body.
- Place ice on the sting site at once; then immerse the sting area in ice water. Remove the tourniquet within five minutes, but keep the sting area immersed for two hours if a doctor cannot be reached. Be sure the ice

138

water extends over the body area well above the sting wound.

- Most important, *get the victim to a doctor immediately.*
- If one must travel in scorpion country, the training guide of the United States Public Health Service recommends taking along a pressurized container of ethyl chloride. It cools the sting site and thus slows down the absorption of venom.

Emergency medical treatment:

- Fortunately, there are antivenoms for the poisonous scorpion species.
- If breathing difficulties develop, calcium gluconate is to be administered, and also artificial respiration if necessary. Sedation can lessen the intensity of convulsions, but some analgesics, such as codeine, morphine and morphine derivitives, may actually increase the toxicity of scorpion venom. Pain in the sting area is thus best treated with Xylocaine. Medical supervision should continue for at least forty-eight hours following the scorpion sting.

What to do if bitten by a centipede:

Disinfect the area and consult a physician.

How to keep from being bitten or stung:

- Remove trash piles, rock piles, lumber piles, discarded mattresses, cardboard, and the like from the area around the home.
- Chickens, ducks, and geese are great scorpion hunters and therefore act as deterrents.
- Crankcase or fuel oil, liberally applied near the home and outbuildings, will discourage scorpions from the vicinity.

TARANTULAS, SCORPIONS AND CENTIPEDES

- Rock walls, stumps, tree trunks, and the like can be treated with an insecticide.
- Arcas inside the home, such as window frames, door-jambs, and baseboards, should also be sprayed to kill scorpions and to discourage their entry.
- Sandboxes should not be provided for youngsters in areas where there are known to be scorpions, since they are a preferred scorpion habitat.
- Wear gloves when handling trash and rubbish piles, stacked lumber, and the like.
- Shake out long-stored clothing and bedding before use. In scorpion country even well-screened homes are occasionally invaded.
- It is interesting to note that in one scorpion-control program in Brazil small boxes were constructed of black paper and placed around the walls of the rooms inside the houses. Scorpions that wandered at night sought the boxes during the day as hiding places. Powerful insecticides were sprayed around the little boxes to kill the scorpions as they moved through to the dark little shelters. According to the account, this simple program was 100 percent effective.

12

From the Mighty to the Mite

Mites and ticks are so closely related as to be kissing cousins. Both are also related to spiders and scorpions and even to that weird flotsam of the beach, the horseshoe crab. All are members of the Arachnida class. Mites and ticks belong to the same order, the Acarina, which, like most other members of Arachnida, predigest their meals outside their bodies, then suck in the resulting mush.

Mites are everywhere: on land, in water, on plants, on animals, and on man. Some thirty thousand different species have been identified, and more are found all the time. More than half the mite species spend at least a part of their lives as parasites and can transfer from one host to another. They can be found on birds, rodents, reptiles, mammals, and even on other insects. For example, one interesting little mite lives and loves in the ear of a moth. It is possible that the reader was unaware that moths have ears. They do, two of them, and they are exceedingly sensitive instruments of hearing. A moth's very survival depends upon its ability to detect the locator pulses of an oncoming bat. A single mite that settles within a moth's ear can produce a lively household within days. The mites puncture the ear membranes to obtain food and soon cost the moth its hearing in the ear. The odd thing is that the mites do not stray to the other ear even when their home becomes vastly overcrowded. It is as if they knew that, if they deafened both ears, the moth would be helpless to escape the bat, and they would accompany it to oblivion down the bat's gullet. One ear, it seems, is enough to give the moth a fighting chance of escaping the bat. How the tiny mites have deduced this is one of those curious and unanswered puzzles that continue to challenge us the more we know about the workings of life on our earth.

Mites range in size from giants of about half an inch to varieties that are invisible to the naked eye and make their presence known only by the itch and the red spots that they produce. It is the minuteness of most of the mite species that makes mite infestation so difficult for the physician to identify, much less treat. A magnifying glass is a great help in locating the culprit, and I keep one in each treatment room just for the purpose of tracking an all-but-invisible mite on a patient's skin. Another aid to diagnosis is the grouping and the location of the bites on the skin. Those are often a dead giveaway in identifying what sort of mite is at work. Occasionally the physician may retrieve the mite with the tip of a lancet or a pencil. He must be careful not to obliterate the beast in the process, and once captured, it must be preserved quickly lest it dry up and disappear. It may be embalmed in a 70 percent solution of alcohol, then studied under a microscope for identification.

Perhaps because mites tend to be so difficult to see, there is such a thing as psychological infestation. The power of suggestion can be powerful enough to make the skin itch and to produce the sensation of "something" crawling. Sometimes the physician will confirm the presence of "bugs" with his magnifying glass, but sometimes too the bugs are all in the patient's head. Being afflicted by the unseen tends to sway the imagination, as I have noted on many occasions when I have lectured on allergy to insects. A good many individuals in my audience begin to scratch after a bit, mildly at first but with increasing intensity, as I discuss symptoms of such insect problems as fleas, lice, scabies, and the like. By the time I have gotten to the subject of mites my audience has usually become very active. This is as true of an audience of physicians as it is of laymen, although I sometimes suspect that at least a few of the scratchers are trifling with the seriousness of my discussion.

One of the best-known mites is the chigger. It lurks in the long grass and brush in summer and launches itself upon us and other animals for its meals. Blackberry pickers know it well, since blackberry canes are one of its favorite launching pads. The common brand of chigger can be found almost everywhere in the United States, although some of the far-western states appear to be free of it. The bright-red chigger larvae can make pure misery of the aftermath of an outing in a daisy-strewn meadow or a hike in the wilds. The adult chigger lives peaceably on vegetable matter, but the larvae must have a blood meal in order to reach maturity. They prefer a chicken or some other animal, but if none happens along, they will take a bite of a human being.

Seen under a microscope, chigger larvae are monsters worthy of any horror movie. Hairy of body, the larvae possess six legs, claws, knifelike jaws, and two pairs of eyes. They emerge from pale-orange, all-but-invisible eggs, of which the chigger lays about three or four hundred in moist earth. As soon as they hatch, the larvae begin a vigorous search for their blood meal. They scurry about grass tops and brush waiting for a warm-blooded animal to come along. When such a host passes by, they clamber aboard. If the host is human, they usually board by way of the feet and work their way upward. When they come to an obstacle of clothing, such as boots, shoes, socks, the belt, or the collar, they attach themselves firmly and settle down to the meal that is vital for their survival. As I said earlier, without blood they cannot move into the next stage of their development as a nymph.

If the human host happens to be sitting or reclining in the lush grass of summer, perhaps to admire the parade of clouds across the sky or to whisper sweet nothings in a beloved's ear, the chiggers are likely to attack the upper torso. Generally, though, they hit below the belt, and chigger bites are most frequently found about the ankles and on the legs. They also

143

often choose the beltline, perhaps because they are stopped there by a reasonably tight belt or perhaps because the waist is relatively tender.

Despite the popular notion that chiggers burrow into the skin, they actually simply attach themselves with their odd jaw claws, called mandibular claws, which not only allow them access to tenderer tissue beneath the outer surface of the skin but also give them a firm anchorage on their victims. Once attached, the chigger secretes a digestive substance that liquifies the cells of the host's epidermis. The chigger then sucks up the resulting fluid. The secretion penetrates deeper and deeper into the skin, liquifying cells on its way and forming a tiny, hollow tube. When the chigger larva has sated its appetite, it drops off the host, usually within three or four days. Unhappily, the secretion that is left behind continues to irritate the skin for quite some time.

Is the host aware when he has picked up these little red devils? Unfortunately, no, not until the chigger is firmly attached and at work liquifying the skin cells. The itch caused by the process of disintegration of one's hide may be the first indication that one is under attack. When the victim traces the itch, he will find a tiny red spot. In the center he may be able to detect the tiny red pinpoint of the larva itself. Within a few hours, or perhaps a day, the red spot becomes somewhat hivelike in appearance, and the itching increases in intensity. Pity the poor woodchuck from which one researcher obtained four thousand chiggers. The animal must have been one huge itch—not much wood could that woodchuck chuck.

As with other insect bites the severe itch often leads to secondary infection, for it takes almost superhuman willpower not to scratch. But if the victim can bear with it and not use his fingernails on the bite itself, both the lesion and the itch usually disappear within a week or so.

There are those who are hypersensitive to the chigger's bite and react to it with marked swelling and deep purple lesions, especially when the bites occur on the legs, abdomen, or genitalia. The genitalia of a small boy are particularly sensitive. Bites there may produce sufficient swelling to interfere with urination. When this happens to a young male patient during the summer months, the doctor can be almost certain that chiggers are the cause. Mild systemic symptoms, such as fever, headache, and general malaise, may also follow chigger bites.

How is a diagnosis made of chigger lesions? The first step is to ask the patient some searching questions. For instance, I might ask a patient sporting such lesions where he has been recently. Out in the fields? The brush? Aha, picking blackberries! I may take a hand lens to the bites, but if the chigger has already eaten and run, this may not clinch the case. The placement of the bites will be a help in diagnosis. As noted earlier, the chigger most often stops and dines where clothing barriers exist. Thus bites around the ankles above the shoe or sock tops, around the beltline, or about the collar or sleeve cuffs are suspect. Also the intense itching and the absence of burrows both indicate the chigger as the culprit.

While our kind of chigger in the United States is more a nuisance than a threat to health, its cousins in other areas of the world are considered dangerous. In Japan and many other areas of Southeast Asia the chigger, along with two other species of mite, is a vector for scrub typhus, a disease that is often fatal. American soldiers in the Pacific theater during World War II suffered almost as much from this disease as they did from malaria, and they feared it more because the mortality rate often ran as high as 5 percent.

Far worse than our brand of chigger in North America are the sarcoptiform mites, better known as the itch mite or scabies. There are various kinds, each of which exhibits a decided preference for one kind of animal host. Some prefer man. Others prefer dogs and man's other domesticated beasts and cause the mange or scab. Some prefer birds, dwelling on and between their feathers. One kind has defined its preferences more sharply and dwells only on the feet of birds.

Acarus scabiei likes human beings. For a long time it was thought that it got its main chance at us only during times of stress and poor hygiene, for instance, during wartime or famine, when people tend to crowd together. During World

145

War II the British were tortured by a full-scale outbreak of scabies when they sought safety in droves in the London tube and other air-raid shelters. Lately scabies has become prevalent again, especially among schoolchildren and, to their embarrassment, among some of their teachers. The children bring it home, and once one family member turns up with the itch mite, it is almost certain that the rest of the family will be afflicted. Transmission of the mites is generally by skin-to-skin contact, although they can be acquired through an exchange of clothing or bedding.

Like the chigger, the scabies, or itch mite, looks horrible under a microscope. Pearl gray or pink in color, it is equipped with four pairs of stubby legs that are bottomed off with claws and with stiff hairs and small spines. Venomous glands open into the mouth area. Fortunately, neither the male nor the female scabies mite lives for long: he departs this life right after mating; she follows him just after laying her eggs, although that can take her several months. The human itch mite burrows into the skin, preferring areas of the body where the skin is thin, for example, between the fingers, in the bends of the elbows and the knees, around the shoulder blades and nipples, and on the penis. The tender skin of the face and scalp of infants may also be infested. The victim is not immediately aware that he is under attack, for it takes about three or four months for sensitization to take place. During this time the female mites are burrowing away, laying a few eggs every two or three days in the burrows. The eggs begin to hatch in about five days, which makes for a lot of unseen activity under the victim's skin.

These young mites develop through four stages from egg to adult. When the mite larva hatches from the egg, it makes its way out of the burrow to the surface of the host's skin. Here it molts several times to become a nymph with eight legs. As a nymph it resides in the crusts of the skin, particularly in the vicinity of hair follicles. After another molt it becomes an adolescent mite, and after a final molt, an adult. Then it mates and, if it is a female, burrows back into the skin to lay eggs to start the cycle all over again. The male goes off to die after mating, his duty done.

The thought of all this activity is enough to make one's skin crawl, which, of course, is what is happening. Yet, as I said earlier, the victim is usually unaware of all the bustle and stir at first. All of a sudden he will begin to itch and to wonder what is getting to him. Reinfested individuals, already sensitized to the scabies mite's secretions, enjoy no such period of grace but begin scratching within hours of the first burrowing.

The itch is the prime symptom of scabies infestation. It is severe and tends to be much worse at night. Small blisterlike vesicles or pimples may form, appearing as a rash, and vigorous scratching may cause them to weep and bleed, making a mess of the victim's skin. Secondary infection then becomes a good possibility.

How is scabies infestation diagnosed? I usually begin by asking if anyone else in the family is suffering from an itch and rash. If the itching is worse at night, this is a characteristic of scabies. I may take a hand lens to see if burrows are present. If they are, I can pick up a female mite with a needle. Once it is under a microscope, there is no doubt about what is going on in the patient's skin.

The animal scabies mite that produces mange rarely transfers itself to human beings. Thus we need not fear the mangy dog, although we may pity him. When mange mites do become parasites on people, they do not remain long. They do not seem to care for what a human host can offer in the way of habitat and sustenance. During their short stay they still can create lesions and itching, although they do not appear to burrow into the skin the way human scabies mites do. Nor is there an initial itch-free sensitization period.

Chicken mites may also briefly transfer their attentions to man, but they too do not stay for long. Bird mites may take up residence with human hosts when their preferred habitat and diet are not available. Rat and mouse mites will accept human beings and other warm-blooded animals, and sometimes the resulting dermatitis is a medical problem in rat-infested cities. There is evidence that they transmit rickettsialpox, a typhuslike disease that has shown up in such rodent-harboring cities as New York and Boston. Sometimes it seems impossible to win in the battle against disease: when rats are eliminated, the attacks of their mites on men intensifies as the starving mites seek a meal anywhere they can find it.

The grain-itch, straw-itch, or hay-itch mite, as it is variously called, attacks both man and animals. It derives its names from its preferred habitats, grain, straw, hay, and grasses. Infestation from these mites was more common in the old days of straw-filled mattresses, but it is still found among grain threshers and others who handle grain. A few years ago a group of young fellows showing their livestock at a country fair came down with the grain itch after they had slept in the straw to be near their animals.

The grain-itch mite causes intense itching, which usually begins about ten hours after it begins to feed. Its bite is a raised, reddened, pimplelike lesion, which quickly forms a small blister filled with purulent fluid. The itching is so bad that secondary infection frequently occurs because of the victim's desperate scratching. Generalized systemic reactions, including fever, headache, and nausea, have also been reported. More commonly, both itch and lesions subside within a few days.

A number of the different mites take up their abode in our edibles. The grain mite not only inhabits our grains but also may be found in cheese and in the vanilla pod. Dock workers handling cheeses may come down with the great itch, and workers with vanilla suffer a dermatitis called vanillism. Another very tiny mite favors not only grain but also dried meats, hams, dried fruits, and collections of dried butterflies and other insects. Obviously its tastes are catholic. Another mite, which inhabits dried fruits, skin, feathers, and other organic materials, causes grocer's itch among those who handle such things. This mite may be lurking in both stores and homes. The tiny mushroom mite also causes an allergic dermatitis of a mixed rash and pimplelike eruption. It too lives in cheeses, dried meat, cereals, and other foods besides mushrooms.

Obviously mites are everywhere and in just about everything we come in contact with during our daily rounds. The most ubiquitous mite of all, however, and the one that has the greatest effect on human health is the house-dust *mite*. So much has been written lately about this invisible dweller in our homes that I shall deal with it in a separate chapter. When I am done, no housewife will ever rest easy again.

READER'S GUIDE TO MITES:

Know the enemy:

- The chigger larva may be seen as a tiny red spot or pinpoint in or around the center of the reddened area of the bite. **(See Plate 24.)**
- To see the scabies mite a hand lens or magnifying glass is needed. The tiny female adult mite is gray or pink. Her burrows are visible to the naked eye, especially on the tenderer skin of children. They appear as whitish, threadlike zigzag marks.

What to do if bitten by a chigger:

Home treatment:
Relief of the itching and prevention of secondary infection are the twin goals of home treatment. Starch baths before bedtime, calamine lotion, and Caligesic ointment are standard measures to relieve the itching. An oral antihistamine, such as Trimeprazine Tartrate, may also be helpful. If the chigger is still present, it should be removed with a needlepoint. When youngsters are the victims, their fingernails should be cut short to help prevent secondary infection from scratching.

149

Doctor's care:
A doctor should be consulted if signs of secondary infection develop, if marked discoloration of the skin or swelling occurs, or if systemic-reaction symptoms are exhibited. **(See Appendix A.)**

What to do about scabies infestation:

Home treatment:
It takes some effort to rid the patient and his clothing and bedding of the scabies mite. Underwear, nightwear, and bedding should be changed every day for at least four days to prevent reinfestation. Other members of the family should be inspected, for many a patient gets rid of scabies only to become reinfested because the mite is circulating the family. The contaminated bedding and clothing of all those affected should be sterilized.

Doctor's care:
A doctor should be consulted because medications to rid the patient of scabies must be prescribed and treatment must be supervised. The physician may prescribe a special cream, or lotion, to be applied over the affected areas after a thorough hot bath or shower, in which liberal amounts of soap are to be used. The medication, which contains the insecticide lindane, should be left on the skin for twenty-four hours. Then another hot, soapy bath or shower should be taken to wash it away. Further applications are seldom necessary, but if they are, they may be made again at weekly intervals.

There are several other methods of treatment, such as the use of sulfur ointment or benzyl benzoate. Repeated applications of the sulfur are usually required, but one application of benzyl benzoate normally does the trick. It literally can be painted over the body from the neck down.

The patient should not be discouraged if both the

itching and the lesions persist for a while, since the treatment itself may cause contact dermatitis.

How to avoid being infested by chiggers:

You probably cannot avoid chiggers if you are a lover of the summer out-of-doors, but you may be able to cut down the frequency and quantity of chigger bites by avoiding tall grass, brush, and especially blackberry thickets. You can try wearing clothing that fits snugly at the collar, wrists, and ankles but is loose everywhere else in order not to provide ideal feeding sites. If you are camping, a cot off the ground is a good deal safer than a sleeping bag on the ground. And lying about in the grass in dreamy indolence is an open invitation to bloodthirsty chigger larvae.

Some repellents are effective, especially those that contain diethyltoluamide (Deet for short). Deet may safely be applied directly to the skin, so repellents containing it can be doused on all exposed parts of the body. For individuals who are sensitive to repeated applications of repellents, powdered sulfur, dusted on the lower parts of the body, is effective for several days. Clothing can be impregnated with a 5 percent solution of a repellent, but, of course, the magic vanishes when the garments are washed or when the wearer gets caught out in a downpour.

The problem of treating a whole area for chiggers with an insecticide is somewhat difficult since the larvae spread out fairly widely in their search for blood. They may infest one part of an area heavily and be nonexistent in another. How do you know where the all-but-invisible chiggers are in residence? Simply take a piece of black cardboard and set it on edge wherever you suspect chiggers abound. In a few minutes, if they are present, they will crawl up the cardboard, and you will find them in clumps on the top edge.

Once you have the chiggers' home country pinpointed, you can treat the infested area with an insecticide.

According to the United States Department of Agriculture, Malathion and lindane are the most effective. If you are against such a move for ecological reasons, you can prevent chigger ambushes by cutting down tall grass, brush, and blackberry canes. If you are fortunate, the chiggers will move out of your area, and you can hope that they will take up with the rabbits or opossums instead.

How to avoid scabies infestation:

The only way to avoid the scabies mite is to avoid close contact with individuals who have scabies. As noted, once scabies gets into a family, most members of the family will become infested. Throughout the world scabies comes and goes in cycles. At the moment we are experiencing a scabies outbreak in the United States, and the mite is busy making life miserable for a good many people. Parents might do well to make periodic checks of their children, particularly those of school age.

13
The House-Dust Mite

Until recently few physicians had ever heard of the house-dust mite. Yet this tiny creature, invisible to the naked eye, is just about everywhere that the climate is at all humid. It is said that the house-dust mite is a descendent of the nest-infesting mite, which somewhere in its evolution discovered the nests of mankind and took up habitation there. Housewives would be horrified if they knew the quantity of mites that their spotless homes can breed, especially in the bedrooms. It is probably just as well that they cannot be seen: women everywhere might just lay down their vacuum cleaners, throw out their dust cloths, and flee their mite-ridden homes. In any case, there is probably no escape except evacuation to a hospital, where mite populations are either very low or nonexistent, or to a desert, where lack of humidity guarantees that mites cannot survive.

The invisible house-dust mite is plump, with short legs. It resembles in miniature a sated tick that has just dropped off a dog. It subsists on human skin scales, and for this reason huge colonies may be found in mattresses and other furniture where human beings spend a good deal of time. It also obtains necessary moisture from proximity to human beings, absorbing what we transpire. Its habitat is dust particles of human and animal dander; kapok and cotton linter shed by furniture, drapes, rugs, and the like; feather particles from pillows; dry rot from the wood of the house itself; and, I suppose, whatever else floats or is tramped into the house. Dust mites are in the ordinary fuzz that the housewife is dismayed to find on her floors, in the dust on furniture tops, in the unseen dust in beds and upholstered furniture. Even foam-rubber mattresses, which allergists thought were allergen-free, have been found to harbor the house-dust mite.

Dust examined under a microscope may show only a few mites or as many as two hundred to one-tenth gram. Thus a whole colony can ride piggyback on a dust particle. The next time the reader enjoys the sight of dust motes dancing up a sunbeam, he can imagine all the tiny goings-on of a mite microcosm riding that beam of light. He, or she, should be aware that, dead or alive, those mites can cause an allergic reaction in the sensitive. The dust mite does not bite or sting; it is not venomous; but in its countless numbers it can be a hazard to human health.

Two species of house-dust mites which appear to be the most numerous inhabitants of our homes have been identified and labeled. Europeans have their own variety (which is also found widely in this country), and we have ours: *Dermatophagoides pteronyssinus* is Old World, while *Dermatophagoides farinae* is our native breed. Researchers on both sides of the Atlantic and, in Asia and Africa have been intrigued by the house-dust mites, and a great many studies of the mites themselves and of their effect on us, their none-too-willing hosts, have been conducted in the last five or six years. It was found that within the home the mites tend to congregate in those rooms most used by the human inhabitants and in the furniture that is most employed. Unfortunately for father, that overstuffed recliner he so dearly loves to occupy on weekends during whole afternoons of televised baseball/or football is probably loaded with house-dust mites. The more he sits in it, the more skin-flake food and vapor he offers to his chair's teeming colony. The mattresses we sleep on are probably even worse, supporting a whole world within a world. And it may be unsettling to the housewife to know

that when she flaps those sheets so energetically on her morning bed-making rounds she is flipping human skin flakes with
hundreds of mites, mite corpses, and mite excreta into the air.

It is even more unsettling to learn the role of the air currents that we establish about our bodies. The air flow rises to
a plume above our heads, and this flow of air is loaded with
debris-dust particles, human and animal dander, and those
mites. We inhale some of all this motley mixture as it moves
steadily past our noses. For those of us who are hypersensitive
to allergens in the environment, this can mean perennial
rhinitis and even asthma, often of considerable severity. In
Chapter 21 we shall see that the house-dust mite is not the
only insect that sandbags some of us as we simply breathe to
stay alive.)

For some time there was speculation about exactly what it
is in dust that causes the allergic reactions of rhinitis and
asthma. Whenever the air grows dusty, many people sneeze
and cough, and some suffer full-scale respiratory symptoms.
It was not until about 1964 that the finger of suspicion
pointed to the mites. A study at that time by Dutch researchers demonstrated a correlation between symptoms of
allergic respiratory reaction to dust and the mite populations
in that dust. They also discovered that both the symptoms of
allergic reaction to dust and the number of mites in residence
rise and fall in a seasonal pattern that coincides with humid
weather. In many places mite populations increase in the fall
and early winter, fall off later when homes are heated and
thus somewhat drier, and fall off during the dry heat of summer. A damp spring brings a resurgence.

Within the home, studies have demonstrated that dust collected from mattresses has the highest concentrations of
mites while dust on the floors contains a good many of the
somewhat dried carcasses of the mites that have succumbed,
presumably to old age or to a dry spell. Moisture is essential
to mites' good health. They take it in with their daily fare of
dander and metabolize it, and they also can absorb it from
the air. By the same token they are always losing water and
must strike a balance between what is gained and what is lost

to stay alive. Studies indicate that relative humidity must stand as high as 70 percent during at least some part of the day for the mites to be able to maintain the necessary balance. Higher temperatures also play a limited role, in dessicating mites. Lowering the relative humidity to 40 or 50 percent and raising the temperature for a period of time should at least reduce house-dust mite populations within the home. Switzerland, with its high-mountain cold, dry air, harbors few mites, for instance, whereas foggy England is aswarm with them.

Researchers in nations all over the world have been busy collecting samples of their house dust to count the teeming populations in it. The results of the shaking of dust bags and the peering into microscopes confirm that the house-dust mite is almost everywhere in some form or other and that it prefers climates where humidity is high and temperatures are moderate.

No one has accused the house-dust mite of transmitting disease to humans. So far the sole indictment against these tiny residents within our homes is that they are highly allergenic and the cause of a good deal of allergic rhinitis and asthma. The symptoms of allergic rhinitis are similar to those of a cold. The sufferer sneezes, sniffles, may have a frontal headache, and generally has a headful. Allergic rhinitis, however, is often more than a cold in that it can lead to other, sometimes more serious, difficulties. The allergic reaction of swelling of the mucous membranes can block proper drainage of the sinuses so that infection or sinusitis results. If the allergic rhinitis is not relieved by treatment or by avoidance measures, middle-ear problems may develop, and hearing may be impaired either temporarily or permanently. But the most serious complication is the development of asthma; for asthma can disable and even kill its victims.

Asthma is characterized by obstruction of the airways to the lungs. This occurs because of several factors. Smooth muscles wrapped around the bronchi constrict, narrowing the airways, while at the same time mucous glands swell and pour forth mucus as the membranes lining the airways are irritated, further obstructing the air passages. The patient literally gasps for breath. All this happens when an allergic reaction releases histamine and other substances within the lung's cells. The familiar wheezing of an asthma attack is caused by the victim's effort to expel stale air from the lungs past mucous plugs that have formed in the airways. Asthma is often preceded by a pronounced cough. Coldlike symptoms of rhinitis also often herald an attack. The attacks can be mild and infrequent; they also can be severe and prolonged and require hospitalization.

Thus the house-dust mite, for all its minuteness, can be exceedingly harmful to human health. For example, I recently learned of the case of a teenage boy in England who had suffered severely from bronchial asthma. Antidust measures within his home such as are described at the end of this chapter in the reader's guide, had apparently eliminated his symptoms. Unfortunately, he went off to a school where he was reexposed to dust and the dust mite. He reacted with fatal *status asthmaticus*, a condition that is continuous and sustained and may lead to death by exhaustion, respiratory failure, or the like.

READER'S GUIDE TO HOUSE-DUST MITES:

Know the enemy:

House-dust mites are invisible to the naked eye.

What to do about the house-dust mite:

- Close the windows and doors, turn the heat up to eighty or ninety degrees, turn the humidifier off, if you have one, and thus transform the home into an artificial desert for half a day. House-dust mite populations will be reduced if not eliminated. Infestation will undoubtedly recur reasonably soon, and this procedure must be repeated at intervals. For this reason allergists rarely recommend it.

- Chemical control is possible. One study employing pesticides that were low in toxicity to humans and other mammals indicated that in solutions of 1 percent some products were 100 percent effective within twenty-four hours of application. Other pesticides were only effective on one or the other of the two most common species of house-dust mite or in solutions greater than 1 percent. The use of chemicals of any toxicity as a control measure against insects embodies some hazard, which may be as yet unknown to those who recommend them.

- Physical measures to keep the home as dust-free as possible offer the safest and most long-lasting means to combat the house-dust mite. As we have noted, the mattress appears to be the dust mite's favorite habitat. Thus the bedroom, where most of us spend at least a third of our 24-hour day, is where most of the cleaning energy needs to be expended. Mattresses can be frequently aired and sunned. Plastic covers go a long way in preventing dust-mite colonization. They should be wiped periodically with soapy water. Bedsprings, bedsteads, and the like should be kept free of dust. Rugs in the bedroom should be small enough to go into the washing machine once a week. Curtains or drapes should be of fiberglass, or venetian blinds that can be washed weekly should be used. Bedding, including blankets, should be washed once a week also. No upholstered furniture should be allowed through the bedroom door. Wood or metal chairs are easily kept free of dust and thus of mites.

- The busy housewife may throw up her hands in dismay at the thought, but it is wise to give the bedroom a daily vacuuming. There should be no sweeping and no shaking of bedding or of rugs in the room—no stirring up of dust with its colonies of mites.

The House-Dust Mite

- Of course, all this is neccessary only for those who are sensitive to dust and the mites. If they do not appear to bother anyone in the family, ordinary, less drastic measures to keep the home reasonably free of dust and mites will suffice. But if someone in the family is allergic to dust, the heroic measures above will go a long way to alleviate their symptoms (and will rid the house of tens of thousands of tiny creatures that you cannot see but who are nonetheless sharing your roof with you).

14

The Bloodthirsty Tick

Anyone who has owned a dog of any breed—with the exception perhaps of pooches of the Fifth Avenue type—will surely recognize a tick when he sees one. Ticks are universal and universally unpleasant. Like mites they are members of the order Acarina, so technically they are not insects. Like all other bugs and like the crab and the crayfish, their legs are jointed, and therefore they are members of Arthropoda.

And they are one of the toughest members of the phylum. They appear to be able to regenerate lost parts of themselves and even repair their mouthparts when mutilated. Unfortunately too, predators pay them little attention, and only we human beings seem desirous of doing them in. They apparently are not considered gourmet fare; thus they have few natural enemies. Worse still, they have never considered population control, and they fill their immediate environment, be it a doghouse or a human house, with countless tick progeny.

Some five hundred different species of ticks are scattered about the earth, and there are few places where they do not exist. In general, they play no favorites when it comes to attaching themselves to a host. Almost any animal will do, even snakes and lizards. Groups of them have been reported as drawing as much as two hundred pounds of blood from a single large animal, such as a horse or cow, in one tick season. They are the first-class vampires of the Acarina order.

The three types of ticks most familiar in our land are the American dog tick (as it is commonly called), the Lone Star tick, and the Rocky Mountain tick of mountain-fever infamy. The American dog tick roams the land east of the Rockies and is especially numerous in the central and eastern sections of the country. As its name implies, it is partial to dogs, but it will accept any red-blooded, warm-blooded host—raccoon, fox squirrel, horse, rabbit, and man—if dog is unavailable at the moment of need. The adult ticks are the vampires. They gather around animal trails and human roadsides to wait until a possible meal of any species comes by, then scramble aboard to attach themselves firmly to its hide. The host goes on about its business often unaware that it has been boarded, for the tick bite itself causes no pain. Once securely in place, the tick settles down to feed, taking six to thirteen days to fill up. While both male and female suck blood, only the female becomes grossly distended. When she finally drops off the host, she is not only sated but also mated, for mating takes place during the long dinner hour.

Once off the host, the female waddles a few steps away and begins propagating the species. She simply deposits between four and six thousand eggs on the ground. During warm weather these hatch in about a month, and the tiny larvae lurk about in the grass and underbrush for smaller warm-blooded creatures to come along, a field mouse, for instance, or a rabbit. They scurry aboard such a host, dine a bit, usually for four or five days, then drop off to go through the first molt toward adulthood. This molt brings them to the nymph stage. As nymphs, ticks again wait for smaller animals to come along to provide one more necessary blood meal. This time they dine a little longer before dropping off to molt once again. The last molt carries them into maturity, although it takes quite a while, sometimes as long as three weeks or a month. Ticks have plenty of time. Adults can survive two years without a meal, although they rarely ever have to wait that long.

The Lone Star tick is found mainly in the South and Southwest and down into Mexico. It also is not at all choosy where it dines, and it is found on birds as well as squirrels, cattle, dogs, man, and so on. While its various stages from egg to maturity are similar to those of the dog tick, it differs from them in that both larvae and nymph, along with the adults, will board larger animals, including us. The sated adult female drops off to lay any number of eggs from two to ten thousand. Then, after such an effort, she expires. She has ensured, and then some, the perpetuation of her species.

The Rocky Mountain wood tick is probably the most infamous of the three common tick varieties, at least in the popular mind. The adult lives by choice in the underbrush and waits patiently for its preferred host—cattle. It will eagerly board other larger mammals, however, including man. Once confined mainly to the western part of the United States, it has ridden the rails, so to speak, to all parts of the country, dropping out of cattle cars to fan out along railroad rights-of-way and off cattle trucks into the areas bordering highways. The nymphs of the species hibernate over the winter to wake in the spring starving for blood. They feed voraciously, then drop off to molt to adulthood. One study of the longevity of these ticks and their ability to exist without a meal demonstrated that the larvae are more vulnerable than the other forms and will frequently die within a month or so of hatching if they cannot find a host. Nymphs, however, can starve for a year before succumbing. Adults can go even longer. The adult ticks are the disease vectors because as adults they have arrived at the stage when they are most likely to dine upon human beings. Out in the west, the land of their origin, they spread their fever from early spring until the hot, dry weather of July, when most ticks seek protection from the sun and heat beneath rocks and rotting vegetation. In the cooler climes of the East and at higher altitudes ticks are a factor into August in the spread of Rocky Mountain fever.

Some species of ticks have eyes and eyesight good enough to see the passing shadow of a host and then scurry after it. Others, eyeless, possess powerful sense organs that can find a victim as much as twenty-five feet away. Thus he who sits upon a log or the ground in tick country draws them like a magnet to himself. All unconscious of the excitement he is causing, he sits there, perhaps puffing on his pipe, while from all directions tiny ticks are hurrying, hurrying to dine.

There are over a hundred different types of ticks north of the Mexican border. Once a tick of any type arrives on a host's hide, it clamps down firmly with its recurved teeth, then strengthens its hold with a kind of cementlike secretion that glues it even more firmly in place. Oddly enough, the tick can disengage swiftly when it so desires, but when the host attempts to pull it off, it takes a real tug, and often as not either the tick's mouthparts are left attached to the skin or a hunk of the host's tissue is torn free with the tick. Either contingency is reason enough never to try forcibly to remove a tick from one's skin. If the mouthparts remain, they are difficult to remove and can cause problems, such as infection, for the host. Sometimes nodules form in a delayed reaction to this foreign tissue, and these may persist for many months, even years.

Ticks are first-class disease vectors. The diseases they transmit can be exceedingly serious not only to humans but also to cattle and poultry. Relapsing fever, for instance, occurs not only among the people of Africa but also among their cattle herds. This tick-borne disease is characterized by recurrent high fever, nausea, and accompanying dehydration. Some cases have turned up in this country, and ticks carrying the spirochetes that cause it have been found. The tick is also responsible for several typhuslike diseases, of which Rocky Mountain spotted fever is one. Once fatal, the latter is characterized by fever, bone and muscle pain, and a reddish eruption. Other diseases transmitted by the tick are Q fever, which is confined mainly to Australia; an encephalitis in Russia; tularemia; and a somewhat mild fever called Colorado fever in our own West. According to a recent report from the Center for Disease Control in Atlanta, Georgia, this last disease has been transmitted in an unusual way. A blood donor became ill shortly after donating a unit of blood. A few days before giving the blood, the donor had removed a tick from his body.

The blood he gave was administered to a man recovering from an operation, and he too came down with Colorado tick fever. A bit of detective work discovered the virus in the serum remaining in the tubing used to transfer the donor's contaminated blood.

Rocky Mountain spotted fever was once pretty well confined to the West, where, oddly enough, more men than women were its victims. Now it is carried by the dog tick in the East, and more women and children than men suffer from it. The virulent disease was first known in Montana and was sometimes called the "black fever" or "black measles" because of the profuse, dark-reddish spots over the skin, which occur especially on the wrists and ankles and sometimes on the back. We should note that Colorado tick fever exhibits many of the same symptoms of fever and bone and muscle pain, but there is no accompanying rash, and the fever is generally milder. Army surgeons stationed at lonely Rocky Mountain outposts in the nineteenth century mentioned the two fevers as one in their reports. The role of the tick in both diseases was not recognized until almost a century later.

Ticks transmit disease differently from mosquitoes and other insects which bite an infected person, and then carry the bacteria or virus to an uninfected individual. The ticks transmit disease from generation to generation through the egg. The female tick becomes engorged on the blood of a relapsing fever victim. She then drops off, lays her eggs, and dies without biting again. The spirochetes, responsible for the disease live on within the eggs, and the tick larvae that hatch carry the infection. When they next bite a human being, relapsing fever may result. So it is with Rocky Mountain spotted fever and other disease.

Besides being carriers of infectious diseases, ticks can produce several miserable conditions in human hosts. Tick-bite granuloma (tumor or growth) can occur days or even months after the bite even though all visible mouthparts have been removed. It is uncertain whether the cause of these tumors is the host's reaction to microscopic pieces of the tick's biting

apparatus left in the wound or a reaction to some toxic substance in the tick's salivary secretions. Whatever the cause,
the growths are not malignant, and they often disappear of
their own accord within a few months. While they persist
they can be a source of anxiety to patient and physician alike
since they resemble the tumors of Hodgkin's disease, lym-
phoma of the skin, or other serious possibilities. In a few rare
cases, when the growths persist for many months or greatly
enlarge, it is sometimes necessary to remove them surgically.
Biopsy, of course, will determine whether or not such tumors
are malignant, and a careful examination of biopsied tissue
might even reveal the presence of mouthparts. It is thought
that such tumors persist and enlarge because of some
stimulating property the tick secretes which retains strength
over a long period of time. The cyst or cone produced by this
irritant is surrounded by a continuing growth of skin cells.
When this cone is removed, the nodules regress to leave little
scarring.

An even stranger and potentially fatal problem, tick
paralysis, may develop from the bite of a tick, especially if it
occurs in the neck area. This condition, painless and feverless
in its early stages, is believed to be caused by toxins secreted
in the female tick's saliva as she feeds. It is also thought that it
takes five to nine days for her to produce the toxin in sufficient
quantity for it to affect the victim. The paralysis is of an
ascending type, beginning in the motor and sensory nerves of
the legs. It ascends progressively and may cause death if it
involves the respiratory system before the tick drops off or is
removed. The paralysis is dramatically relieved when the tick
is removed. Recovery often occurs within twenty-four to
forty-eight hours. Children under two are the most susceptible, but tick-bite paralysis can occur in older children and
adults as well.

Girls tend to suffer this condition more often than boys.
Their hair is usually longer and thus is more likely to conceal
a tick attached in the neck area around the base of the skull or
on the head itself. Wherever ticks are present, children should

be carefully inspected during tick season each evening before they go to bed, and the area of the neck and the head should receive the closest scrutiny.

Early symptoms of tick paralysis commonly are irritability, general malaise, and loss of appetite. The paralysis itself becomes manifest a day later. Removal of the tick presents something of a problem; for, as we have noted, the trick is to get it off intact lest the mouthparts remain embedded to cause further trouble. The youngster or any person who has just suffered from tick paralysis needs nothing more to contend with.

Another possibility has just recently come under investigation; ticks may carry a virus that causes a form of arthritis. More than fifty people, most of them children, were somewhat abruptly stricken with the illness within a time span of a few years. All the victims lived in a cluster of three small towns in Connecticut. First discovered in Lyme, the virus was dubbed "Lyme arthritis," and as such created widespread interest in the medical profession. The disease is characterized by headache, weakness, usually some fever, general malaise, and pain and swelling in one or more joints, most frequently including the knee. While most attacks last only a week or so and are generally mild, some victims have ended up at least temporarily in wheelchairs. Between attacks the patients enjoy complete remission, and such symptom-free periods can last anywhere from several months to a year or more. It has been reported that, since the disease was first noted, some of its victims have suffered as many as four episodes.

Ticks are under suspicion for several reasons. Many of the patients reported that they suffered a large, round lesion about a month before the arthritis symptoms appeared. The lesions that they described were similar to the kind sometimes caused by tick bites. The disease is occurring among people living in sparsely setted wooded areas where ticks are common. There is also a seasonal pattern, with three-quarters of the patients demonstrating symptoms during the summer or early autumn.

The Bloodthirsty Tick

No one is yet certain about the causes of Lyme arthritis, and a good deal of research is under way. Some arthritis specialists, who have long suspected that a virus might be the cause of other forms of this often crippling disease, are watching the investigation with great interest and with the hope that it may provide an important breakthrough in understanding the disease itself.

READER'S GUIDE TO TICKS:

Know the enemy:

There are soft-bodied ticks that feed rapidly on human beings much as bedbugs do. But the ticks that we are most familiar with are flat and hard-bodied, with six legs in the larva stage and eight in the adult. When engorged, the female is grayish in color and can be as large as half an inch in size. **(See Plate 25.)**

How to remove a tick intact:

A drop of gasoline, kerosine, benzine, alcohol, or ether on the general region of the tick's head will make it loosen its grip. So will a lighted match or the tip of a burning cigarette. However, the tick will take its own sweet time releasing its grip, and the host must be patient. It will frequently, be ten minutes or so before the tick drops off, but when it goes, it will take its mouthparts with it. A tick can also be killed by covering it with a drop of paraffin or fingernail polish, for these substances will close the two tiny breathing openings on its sides and suffocate it.

Under no circumstances should an engorged tick be squeezed, for this will only force more toxin into the bite.

TICKS

TICKS

Treatment of a tick bite:

Once the tick is removed, the bite area should be washed with soap and water, and iodine or another antiseptic should be applied. If a growth or granuloma appears at the site, consult your physician just to be sure that no more serious problem arises. Do this also if signs of infection appear in the bite area.

How to avoid being boarded by a tick:

- For the dog lover and outdoors person avoiding ticks is not easy. Marines at Camp Lejeune, North Carolina, took to wearing dog and cat flea collars around their ankles to discourage both the ticks and the chiggers. Marine top brass discouraged the practice because of the hazards of absorption and inhalation of the insecticides used in the collars, but according to one officer, Marines can still be seen on occasion with flea collars circling their legs just above their boots. Wearing long pants and high boots into the field does tend to discourage tick invasion, as will liberal use of repellents containing Deet.

- Dogs will bring ticks into the house and home area, where they are bound to drop off sooner or later and seek nooks and crannies to lay their thousands of eggs. The entrance of a single tick may produce a tick population explosion in the house practically overnight. Therefore dogs should be regularly treated with a tick dip, spray, or powder from early spring to first frost.
  Small children should be examined nightly for ticks, with special attention paid to the head and back of the neck. Adults would do well to undergo the same routine, especially during June and July, the peak tick season.

The Bloodthirsty Tick

- To discover whether ticks infest an area, tie a piece of white flannel to a string and drag it through the grass or underbrush. Examine it frequently. If ticks are present, they will scramble aboard.

- Controlling ticks once they have settled in an area is difficult. Keeping grass mowed and underbrush cut down will discourage them considerably, but they are tough to eradicate—and fecund.

Symptoms of tick-borne diseases to watch out for:

Rocky mountain spotted fever:
Fever, bone and muscle pain, profuse reddish eruptions on the skin, especially around the wrists and the ankles.

Tick-bite granuloma:
Tumorlike swelling at the site of the tick bite.

Tick paralysis:
Irritability, loss of appetite, malaise, paralysis beginning in the legs and ascending.

15

Fleas:
The Blood Siphoners

Fleas belong to the order Siphonaptera, which seems logical since they are perfectly adapted to siphon our blood and the blood of our pets plus that of a host of wild mammals in the field and wood. The agile flea is a bloodsucker par excellence, but it is more than that, and mankind must always take this tiny insect seriously. More than once it has emptied man's greatest cities and filled his graveyards all over the world. It is believed, for instance, that the flea-borne plague which began in Egypt in the sixth century, spread over the Roman empire and into Europe, and lasted half a century before it finally burned out, claimed a hundred million human lives. It is estimated that in the fourteenth century flea-borne black death killed a fourth of the population of Europe. When the rats began dying, people knew that they were next, even though they did not recognize the flea as the instrument of death.

In former times men did not comprehend why the plague appeared in waves, rising to a grim crescendo, then waning until only a few cases were reported for a number of years. We have since discovered several things about the plague and why in recent centuries it has not swept us away in epidemics as it once did. The distinctly seasonal incidence of the disease coincided with weather conditions that were most favorable for fleas. When the world suffered from drought, the fleas suffered with it—to human benefit.

In temperate climates such as Europe's, plague epidemics reached their peaks during the summer months, but in the tropics the hot, dry summer season usually brought an end to an epidemic. Fleas without hosts (rats, cats, dogs, man, and the like) cannot survive if they lose a certain amount of body water content. Thus hot, dry weather can be their undoing. One early experiment demonstrated that an estimated 80 percent of a flea's body weight is water and that, when the water is decreased to about 60 percent, the flea dies.

Hans Zinsser in his fascinating book *Rats, Lice, and History* cited the domestication of rats as a reason why we humans no longer are threatened by plague epidemics. Rats have ceased to wander; they stay put and thus do not carry the plague to neighboring rat and human populations.

When we human beings finally caught on to the association between rats and the plague, we discovered that, if we got rid of the former, we also largely rid ourselves of the latter. As we brought the rat under some control, the plague receded, although now and again sporadic cases rise to haunt us even in our somewhat antiseptic Western world. It is not inconceivable that the plague could strike again in epidemic form, which is why we should wage an unrelenting war against rats in our cities and elsewhere.

Unfortunately, fleas are not too particular about their hosts. Rat, cat, or dog fleas will take on humans if they must, even though in their heart of hearts rat fleas prefer rats; cat fleas, cats; and so on (there is even one flea species whose predilection is for snakes). If hungry enough, fleas will condescend to dine on anything that comes along. Thus, when the rats died first of the plague, the fleas bearing their deadly gift abandoned the carcasses and turned to humans and in this fashion spread the disease from animals to men. For example, during the turn-of-the-century plague epidemic in California, it was found that of a number of fleas captured most were rat and mouse species, and only a few were specific to humans.

California, long a mecca for those seeking a perfect climate, has a flea problem of some magnitude. Climatic conditions are as attractive to fleas as to human beings in much of the state, and high-humidity areas along the coast, where weather extremes are rare, are especially paradise for fleas, as any newcomer to the region soon finds out. There is a story of a man who decided to buy a hardpan ranch to get away from fleas. It was his understanding that, if the ground was impervious enough, the fleas could not survive. He found a suitable bit of land that he could not loosen with a crowbar and purchased the place, called "Ranchos du las Polgas." After he moved in, he called upon a neighbor and was astonished to find that the family lived in a loft; that, in fact, when bedtime came, they left their clothes at the foot of the ladder leading to the loft and climbed as rapidly as they could to their beds, hoping to leave the fleas downstairs for the night. The newcomer could not understand how fleas could live in such soil, but his neighbor assured him that not only did the hardpan land make no difference at all to fleas but the translation of the Spanish for the ranch he had just purchased was "Ranch of the Fleas." The moral of this tale is twofold: fleas cannot care less about the condition of the soil, since it is not their normal habitat, and before buying a ranch with a Spanish title, be sure you understand a little Spanish.

It seems strange that anything as small and insignificant as a flea could almost bring human civilization down and, in fact, did bring it to a standstill, if not regression, more than once. A flea is small and flat, covered with a hard exoskeleton. When magnified, it somewhat resembles a grasshopper run over by a steamroller. It is hardy and cannot be squashed or slapped out of existence. It derives its phenomenal agility from its highly developed posterior legs. Long and slender, they give the flea a froglike leaping power. Cameras have caught the almost incredible broad-high jump of the tiny creature, demonstrating that it can leap almost a foot straight up and over a foot forward. As it leaps, claws on all six legs are extended forwards to act as tiny grappling irons or landing gear. When it launches itself at an intended victim, it is ready for action the minute it lands. It has even been suggested that the flea can make several somersaults in the air and land right side up on the intended host. Its piercing and sucking mouthparts are ideally suited to dining on blood. All in all, the flea is feisty and formidable.

The flea's life cycle runs the course of a complete metamorphosis from egg to larva to pupa to adult, and it is only the adult form that parasitizes warm-blooded animals (and snakes and the like). The legless larvae usually dwell in the beds, lairs, nests, and homes of the adult fleas' hosts, subsisting on dried blood and animal debris left behind by the unwitting inhabitants. During the pupal stage the immature flea may stay wrapped in its cocoon for many months, waiting patiently, we can suppose, for dinner to come along. A family that includes its pet in its vacation plans is likely to return to a house alive with an eager flea population that has exploded in their absence. Flea eggs left behind will have hatched, and the fleas will have completed their metamorphosis, ready as adults to confront the returning residents. And they will be hungry. With the dog gone on vacation, they will have lost their meal ticket and, famished, will not be too finicky about who provides the blood, dog or human beings.

The whole cycle can vary considerably, depending for the most part on environmental conditions. It can take place in as brief a time as eighteen days or as long a time as twenty months. Under ideal conditions the flea eggs hatch, and the larvae and pupae move through their stages rapidly, as though eager to grow up and have the chance to dine upon some warm, furry creature or an accommodating human being.

How the flea larva emerges from the egg is interesting. A restless creature all of its leaping life, it tumbles about even at this early age within the shell until a sharp spine in the area of its head cuts through the shell to release it. The yellowish-white maggotlike larva emerges, destined to harry whatever suits its dietary fancy.

There are about one thousand flea species, and while they differ somewhat in anatomical configurations, they all live much the same sort of life. Some of them can inflict gruesome

173

damage on human beings, besides being carriers of the plague and typhus. The smallest of fleas is the jigger flea, often called sand flea or chigoe (not to be confused with the chigger). Once on human skin, this tiny tropical species burrows and, if it is a gravid female, will swell to the size of a seed pea. When egg-laying time comes, the flea pops the eggs out through a hole in the host's skin and then dies. In the meantime her burrowing and swelling causes both intense itching and somewhat severe pain. The cyst that results often becomes infected, and the unfortunate host can die of gangrene or tetanus. Since the flea prefers to burrow in the feet and ankles and particularly under the toenails, it is easy for infection to occur. Unfortunately, this flea, which was once confined to our hemisphere, has now been transported across the oceans to Africa and Asia, where it has caused extensive suffering.

The sticktight flea is more irritating than dangerous. It is so named because it attaches itself in one spot on its host rather than jumping from one meal to another. It is especially fond of gathering on the heads of chickens and in the ears of small animals such as rabbits, cats, and dogs. It also likes the area of the eyes, and its bites and the ulcers that they can create may lead to blindness.

Human beings have their own brand of flea, called *Pulex irritans*. It prefers us above all, but like other fleas, its tastes are catholic, and it will settle for a dog or a cat or the like if it must. It has adapted to us nicely. It accepts our clothing as a residence in lieu of fur. Instead of the debris found in dens or nests, the larvae make do for their subsistence with what they can find around our houses. Any kind of organic waste will provide them with food. Thus cleanliness not only is next to godliness but also tends to be next to flealessness.

What happens when a flea bites? Actually, it does not bite so much as it saws the skin open with its rather specialized equipment, which consists of several stylets. Then it draws up the blood, or pumps it out, from the wound. It is not content with one spot and moves restlessly about the host, feeding now here, now there. Thus a single flea can be responsible for a number of itchy bites.

Fleas

Like mosquitoes, fleas find some of us more attractive than others. Frequently within a family only one or two members will serve as hosts while everyone else goes flea-free. Age, sex, and body odor account for flea preference just as they do for mosquito preference. Traditionally women seem to have been the preferred flea victims. Fleas are evidently attracted by sex hormones.

Fleas are a nuisance for many of us and more than a nuisance for those sensitive to the secretions that they inject into their bites. The secretions have a sensitizing effect. Research has demonstrated that initial fleabites cause no noticeable reaction on the skin for a while, but that in a few days sensitivity develops. Even bites that were not marked at first may flare up later and become hard, red, and itchy. A regular pattern has been noted among those who have become sensitized. At first they suffer a delayed reaction as above. Then they go through a period during which they suffer both an immediate and a delayed reaction. Finally, they develop some immunity, and during this period of grace flea bites are again scarcely noticeable. In this manner probably most native Californians have become immune to the state's flea hordes. Newcomers to that sunny state are more likely to complain bitterly about being bitten. Unfortunately, in most climates folks have to go through the whole process of sensitization and immunity over and over again, following the waxing and waning of flea activity that occurs with weather and temperature fluctuations.

Since fleas have a habit of probing about on the skin and dining here and there, the lesions they cause come in groups. The papules can be about the size of a pencil eraser, and often there are three or more fairly close together. I have noticed that they frequently form a Z, like the mark of Zorro. They are most often found on the legs, arms, face, hip, and shoulder areas. Youngsters hugging their new puppy or kitten may demonstrate the results on their necks and chests. In fact, since children commonly play at ground level, they are the most frequent flea victims. Also, during the fleas' most active season youngsters are likely to be wearing a minimum of

175

clothing, thus exposing vast, tempting and tender areas.

That children must often pay the flea piper for its tune is demonstrated by one doctor's case history of a small boy who continually sported spots. It was discovered that the boy's family was in the habit of gathering in the warm kitchen by the stove and that an overstuffed chair there was alive with fleas. Grandmother spent her days comfortably in that chair, and the family cat took over at night. Both grandmother and cat kept the chair warmed and an ideal breeding place for flea mothers to lay their eggs. They maintained a constant diner for flea adults as well.

In general, the worst a fleabite can do is become infected. Since it itches mightily, this is a good possibility, especially among children. But if we controlled the flea for no other reason, it is because typhus and the plague still lurk among us, ready to blossom in our modern world even as they have in past centuries. Sporadic outbursts occur now and again even in the somewhat antiseptic United States. The United States has had more cases in the last several years than during the last half century. In the West plague-bearing fleas have killed many a ground squirrel that served as their host before succumbing. People and their pets may then be fair game for the hungry, disease-ridden fleas.

To end this chapter on a less grim note let me recommend an interesting and amusing discussion of fleas, *The Compleat Flea*, by Brendan Lehane (New York: Viking Press, 1969). I have tried hard not to beg, borrow, or steal any of his fascinating facts, but the temptation was great.

READER'S GUIDE TO FLEAS:

Know the enemy:

The flea is brown, flat, wingless, and hard-bodied with long slender legs. **(See Plate 26.)**

What to do about flea bites:

Home treatment:
Flea bites are generally treated much like chigger bites with anti-itching medications and lotions, including oral antihistamines (for instance, Temaril), starch baths at night, and calamine lotion. The bites should be washed with soap and water, and an antiseptic should be applied to lessen the chances of secondary infection. Youngsters should have their fingernails cut short to prevent infection from the inevitable scratching. On occasion individuals have suffered a systemic reaction to flea bites. **(See Appendix A** for a list of systemic-reaction symptoms.)

Doctor's care:
If signs of infection develop, such as redness, swelling, heat, and pain, a doctor should be consulted. Parents should watch for signs of impetigo following flea bites, for this is a fairly frequent consequence.

How to avoid fleas:

Preventing the invasion of fleas in the home or home environment can be an unending chore for the animal lover. Pets who dwell under the same roof with human beings should be kept as flealess as possible by periodic dusting, spraying, or antiflea bathing. Many of the products on the market are quite effective, but the key to success is to keep it up and to be sure also to treat pet beds and "curling-up" places. The United States Department of Agriculture recommends Malathion, Ronnel, and pyrethrins as insecticides for the spraying of such flea-infested areas as cellars. Vacuuming within the home should be frequent when there are pets in residence, since this is an excellent way to get rid of flea eggs and larvae. For the same reason rugs should be shaken often and washed whenever possible.

Recent studies of oral thiamine chloride as a repellent against such insects as fleas have demonstrated some effectiveness, although conclusive proof has yet to be compiled. It might well be worth consulting your physician about this nontoxic preventive drug if fleas and their bites are a real problem, especially if children are involved.

16

The Lowly Louse

No one knew what it was. It appeared out of nowhere. It began suddenly with a severe headache and back pain. Legs and arms began to ache, and the victims became so weak that they could scarcely move. Within a couple of days fever began ravaging their wracked bodies, and although they had no thermometers to register the 105 degrees, the doctors of the day were appalled by such raging fevers. The tongues of the patients turned white with fur or else totally black, rolling up oddly in the backs of their mouths. Faces became dusky, and on the fourth or fifth day bluish spots would appear on the sufferers' abdomens and other parts of their bodies. The diesease was so often fatal that, when such symptoms developed, families despaired, and physicians shook their heads forebodingly.

What was not comprehended back then in the early sixteenth century was that the lowly louse had become a destroyer. The instrument of its malevolence was epidemic typhus, a cruel and killing disease that can still be fatal in spite of modern antibiotics. Like the flea, the tiny louse almost sent the human race back to the cave. Louse-borne typhus haunted the troops and famine-ridden civilians of World War I. Like monkeys in a cage grooming each other, soldiers used to hunt for lice on comrades and themselves. A

179

cootie hunt could be an occasion to break up the boredom of the trenchs between battles.

There are several thousand different species of lice, but the two that human beings need be most concerned about are body lice (*Pediculus humanus*) and crab lice (*Phthirus pubis*). The so-called head louse is actually a variant strain of the body louse. Both body and crab lice are sucking lice and belong to the order Anoplura. They prefer human beings above all else, but can be transferred to rabbits in the laboratory, which suggests that they will, if they must, seek other mammals as hosts when humankind is not available. In general, different species of lice appear to follow related species of hosts. Thus the body louse is closely related to the louse that loves the primates. It may be that it evolved from a primate louse strain, or vice versa.

Lice are anything but attractive. Gray or dirty white in color, crablike in appearance, with pointed heads and pointed teeth (the better to grip us by), they would win no beauty contests. We have various names for them, none of them distinguished. We call them "cooties" or "graybacks" or "mechanized dandruff" or "seam squirrels" to indicate our contempt.

By whatever undistinguished name it goes by the louse is a pest and a menace. In a way, it may be poetic justice that during recent centuries it has done its worst to the human race when we have not been at our best. During wartime, when human values go astray, and social customs and the rules of law and of love go amok, human hygiene also vanishes, and the louse moves in, delighted with the decline of the human condition. The lice are quick to take advantage of the lack of soap and water, the crowded conditions, the enfeebled, exhausted bodies of the starving and the warring. Lice are passed around by direct body contact or by contaminated bedding or clothing. Unfortunately, they are able to survive a week or so without a meal and so can lie in wait. They are not great travelers but cling closely to their host or his clothing, leaving only if the host himself dies. When sated with blood, they may slip into the folds or seams of his clothing or bedding to relax until hunger strikes again. In the main, however, they like to stay skin-close.

Even the louse eggs are unhandsome. They are small, white or gray, and gluey. The female louse lays them in the fabric of clothing or glues them to the host's body hairs. A human host can harbor as many as five hundred body lice; a single piece of clothing can shelter ten thousand eggs. The hatching of the eggs is somewhat strange. They come equipped with little lids at one end. When the embryo becomes a larva, it swallows a bit of air, then impolitely expels it from its anus. The resulting tiny explosion blows the lid off, and out comes the baby louse. As soon as they have freed themselves from the eggs, the tiny larvae hurry to a meal of blood, wasting no time between the molts that bring them to adulthood. The host provides from egg to adulthood. Since a single female louse lays about three hundred eggs during her short but active life span of three or four weeks, and since she lays between eight and a dozen daily, it is easy to see how a person can be literally crawling with lice during the space of a few short weeks. Unfortunately, the changing seasons bring no relief as they do with some other insect pests. The louse is happy no matter what the weather.

One might think that a malnourished human being would result in malnourished lice, but that is not the case. Lice seem to be even healthier on the unhealthy. Laboratory studies have demonstrated that rabbits with vitamin deficiencies supported lice as well as or better than well-nourished rabbits who were getting vitamins aplenty.

Head lice are usually a little smaller than body lice. They unfortunately possess ability to change color more or less to match the hair in which they nestle, which makes it difficult to detect the adult lice. The eggs glued to a hair shaft, however, are there for all the world to see. Head lice make a mess of one's crowning glory. They most often take up positions at the back of the head, nape of the neck, or around the ears, and can sometimes even be found among the hairs of the eyebrows, eyelashes, and beards. Rather naturally, they prefer the long, thick hair of women and children. When infestation is heavy, the hair can become matted with the gluey eggs, which are called nits; the feeding lice; and the secretions from the pustules or pimples that the lice raise on the scalp. To put it very mildly, the head of an individual who is carrying a load of lice is gruesome.

When lice first take up residence in a person's hair, they are not felt, and the victim remains unaware of their presence. But after they have been around for a week or ten days, the individual becomes sensitized, and his head begins to itch. If infestation continues and the lice become a part of one's life, one develops tolerance to their feeding. In fact, in some parts of the world a healthy colony of lice on one's head testifies to one's virility. In other out-of-the-way places religious taboos make killing a louse a sin, although it is permissible to remove one's louse gently and lay it on a friend, so to speak.

Pubic lice, commonly called crab lice, have heads that are more rounded than those of their body- and head-lice cousins. This does nothing to lessen their repulsiveness. Their forelegs end in large claws, the better to grasp hair with. Thus they resemble miniature crabs. While they are sometimes found in the armpits and even among the hairs of the eyebrows, they mainly confine themselves to the pubic area. Relatively inactive, they tend to remain stationary during their short life span, hanging on with their teeth as they suck blood. They are not quite as prolific as body lice: the female crab louse lays about fifty eggs during her lifetime, just enough to keep things going.

When lice bite, they leave tiny red spots on the skin. At first the spots are flat and even with the skin's surface, which makes them distinct from other insect bites. But shortly the spots become pimple or hivelike, and then they may begin to itch severely. Scratching often causes them to ooze and become crusted and scaly, as in eczema. As we have noted, the victim of lice infestation, or pediculosis, as it is called technically, does not react initially to the presence of his new guests. It takes about a week before the itching begins. Oddly enough, studies have demonstrated that itching and redness frequently appear after this sensitization period in old bites that were symptomless until new areas of the skin were bitten.

Experiments to determine just what it is in the louse's bite that causes inflammatory responses in human skin showed that both louse feces and louse heads contain toxins that can irritate. Individuals who harbor lice for a lengthy period of time develop characteristicly hardened and darkened skin, which is sometimes called "Vagabond's disease."

Lice can also cause systemic symptoms of irritability, weariness, and mental depression. For instance, there is a medical report of a teenage farmhand who became so badly infested and reacted with such severe symptoms of systemic reaction that he had to be hospitalized. The boy, who had hitherto enjoyed superb health, woke one morning with aching, stiff legs and an odd feeling of weakness. Within a day he had developed fever, headache, and a hacking cough. Once he was admitted to the hospital, the lice were discovered, plus the odd discolored patches on the skin that are associated with pubic-lice infestation. The young man was treated—in this case with a copper-salt solution applied to the hairy parts of his body—and within twenty-four hours his fever disappeared, and he felt fine. A day later his temperature rose again, however, and a more careful examination revealed lice remaining on other parts of his body. When these too were eliminated, his temperature returned to normal, and he was soon discharged, his old healthy self with his lice colony gone.

What lice do best, as noted above, is transmit serious epidemic diseases. They have been responsible not only for epidemic typhus but also for epidemics of relapsing fever, an uncomfortable illness characterized by headache, fever, chills, and pains throughout the body. It can be fatal. Lice were also the villains in trench fever, which swept through the armies of World War I and even turned up during World War II in troops in Eastern Europe. A nonfatal disease, it too brings fever, headache, dizziness, and muscle and bone pain. To be infested with lice is not only uncomfortable and repellent but also hazardous.

Early in World War II the United States government recognized the possible hazard of lice-borne disease, especially typhus, and undertook various programs of lice control. Since lice infestation was rare among our citizens, laboratories working on lice-control methods had to find a way to raise and maintain lice colonies for experimentation. At the time the only way they knew to obtain supplies of lice was to have volunteers feed them twice a day. Naturally there was some difficulty in finding people who were willing to feed lice colonies twenty-five to fifty thousand strong on their backs morning and afternoon. Nevertheless, in this manner millions of lice were reared. After each feeding period they were nestled back into bits of cloth and kept pleasantly warm. Their eventual fate, of course, was to be the subjects for tests of various chemical products as investigators tried to find out what would kill them best. One of the resulting products was DDT, which probably saved millions of lives among refugees, concentration-camp survivors, and troops toward the end of the war. Blown up under the clothing with hand dusters, this powerful insecticide not only killed the adult lice but remained potent for so long that any larvae that later hatched also died. Unfortunately, by the time of the Korean War lice had become DDT-resistant, and other chemical means of control had to be found. The recurrent nightmare of scientists who work on such things is that lice will become resistant to all known chemical methods of control. Then we would have no effective weapon against such louse-borne epidemic diseases as typhus and plague.

People who cannot stay clean and who are overcrowded are likely prospects for lice infestation. But even those who practice cleanliness can contract a case of lice, mainly through direct contact with someone who is infested. It is also possible to acquire lice by indirect contact, for instance, by borrowing someone's comb or hairbrush. Blacks seem more resistant to head lice than are whites. It is thought that hair texture may have something to do with this or some difference in the substances secreted by the scalp. Some individuals are much more sensitive to lice saliva than are others. They react with intense itching and much more pronounced lesions. Other people can be literally crawling with the creatures without much noticing their presence. Barbershops and beauty salons where hygiene practices are somewhat slipshod may pass lice around among their customers. Contact can be made in public restrooms. Youngsters in school may provide each other unwittingly with a few lice. Not too far in the past schoolteachers held regular morning head inspections among their other duties.

Lice are all that we have in mind when we denigrate someone we dislike by calling him a louse, or when we characterize something as lousy. Small, mean, repulsive creatures, best avoided by mankind, they are, nevertheless, a part of nature's grand scheme and no doubt here to stay. We must be aware of their existence lest we find that they are existing upon us.

READER'S GUIDE TO LICE:

Know the enemy:

Lice are gray or dirty white in color and tiny in size. (**See Plate 27.**)

What to do about lice infestation:

- Consult your doctor. Effective medications must be prescribed, and since they are likely to be potent, careful instruction in their use is necessary. Lindane ointment, for instance, is effective against body lice. So is an application of benzyl-benzoate emulsion. First comes a good shower with plenty of soap and water, then an application of whatever the physician prescribes.

   Head lice and crab lice are also treated with benzyl benzoate applied to the hair with a brush and followed by a thorough shampooing with soap and water twenty-four hours later. If infestation is heavy, the process may have to be repeated several times. If the host's tresses are long, it would be prudent to adopt a shorter hairdo for awhile, but shaving the head, as was once done, is too drastic and unnecessary.

Areas of secondary infection on the scalp should be treated with antibacterial ointments such as bacitracin or neomycin.

- Bedding and clothing should be boiled.
- Combs and brushes used by the lice-infested should be sterilized. Any head covering or hat used while the victim was playing host should be discarded, or if it can be boiled or treated with benzyl-benzoate emulsion without ruin, it should thus be rendered lice-free.
- The victim's hair should be examined carefully each week for a month or so to be certain that reinfestation has not taken place and that eggs that have survived the above procedures have not hatched to start the whole process over again.

How to prevent lice infestation in the first place:

Good personal hygiene is the key, although it must be emphasized that anyone, no matter how exalted his or her station, can pick up a few lice. Barber shops, beauty parlors, and public rest rooms where hygiene practices may be slipshod can harbor the not-easily-noticed lice. The generous soul who lends a hairbrush or comb among friends is not only inviting lice aboard but perhaps ensuring that he, or she, is not the only victim. The maxim that personal toilet articles are for personal use is a good one.

17
The Ubiquitous Bedbug

About 80 percent of the human race live intimately with bedbugs. One's home need not be a hovel to give them shelter,
and many world travelers have met with them in some of the
poshest hotels. Some of the most regal lodgings of Paris have
been known to harbor whole armies. We define some of our
insect infestations as being beyond the social pale, and as a
physician treating bedbug bites off and on, I have heard the
argument, "We don't have bedbugs. Therefore these cannot
possibly be bedbug bites." It would seem that nice people
simply do not invite the attentions of some insects, bedbugs
among them. Nice people are also never infested by cockroaches, silverfish, lice, or scabies. Fleas, however, become
socially acceptable if one has a cat or dog. Bees, wasps, and
the like suffer no social stigma; anyone can be occasionally
plagued by Hymenoptera. Although we rate our insect pests on
a social scale, it is wise to recall on occasion that there were
bedbugs in practically every bed that George Washington
slept in. He may have been bothered by the creatures, but he
surely attached no stigma to his hosts, since bedbugs were as
universal as flies. In many parts of the world they still are.

One need not be poor or dirty to acquire them. Customs
officials in many lands have discovered bedbugs hitchhiking
a ride in real leather luggage stamped with the owner's ini-

tials in gold. Still, bedbugs thrive where cleanliness is an alien practice, although the tiny, flattened, brownish-red creatures do not arise fully formed from the sweat of the sleeping as Aristotle once proclaimed.

Bedbugs are true bugs and belong to the order of Hemiptera, the "half-wing" insects, so named because most of them have forewings that are half-membranous and half-leathery. Bedbugs are closely related to aphids and other garden pests, such as leaf hoppers, but they subsist on blood rather than plant juice. There are some thirty species, eight of which dwell among us in North America, and one of which dines eagerly on us and our fellow men in Europe. The latter is the ubiquitous *Cimex lectularis,* a flatish creature when not engorged with our life's blood.

Bedbugs possess three pairs of legs, which give them the power to scuttle about for their meals, then disappear down cracks and crannies with the first light of dawn. They are all but wingless, having only vestiges of them. Nocturnal by nature, they hide by day behind such things as baseboards and trim or in bedsteads and emerge at night when dinner climbs into bed. Being gregarious by nature, whole extended families of bedbugs gather in these convenient hideouts to sally forth in small armies to assail their sleeping host. Usually they do not migrate about, but sometimes they are transported, perhaps against their will, in clothing and the like. Generally, once established in someone's bed, they seek no further horizens. They settle down to a comfortable life, dining by night, sleeping by day. If this easy existence is disrupted by the absence of their meal ticket, they may migrate on water pipes or electric wires into someone else's bed.

The bedbug possesses a beaklike proboscis, or sucking tube. It employs this, together with its mouthparts, to make a hole in the host's skin, then probes about in search of a juicy capillary vessel full of blood. Since the bedbug often feeds for as long as five minutes without disturbing the sleep of its host, it is thought that it probably injects a bit of anesthesic into the wound. There is a story of one man who, all unaware, played host to so many bedbugs so often that he became severely anemic. One of the known constituents of the bedbug's salivary secretions is an anticoagulant, which gives it the ability to suck blood for a rather long period undisturbed by clotting.

The bedbug has one feature that makes it different from other household bugs: a pair of stink glands that exude an oily secretion with a characteristically pungent and unpleasant odor. A traveler with a good nose for such things can tell the moment he steps into a room whether it is already occupied.

The bedbug's life cycle starts with an egg. During her life span the female may lay two hundred to five hundred eggs in batches of three or four a day. The eggs are rather large and yellowish-white. Usually they are laid in a small patch. Depending on the temperature, they commonly hatch within a week or so. The emerging bedbug moves at a deliberate pace through five molts to adulthood. Unfortunately for us, it needs a blood meal every step of the way in order to reach maturity. Thus the bedbug that hatches in the bedding is busy from the moment it emerges from the egg until it dies. It may even be active as a carcass because it makes up a part of the house dust that causes housewives to sneeze and brings asthma, especially to children.

Once the bedbug reaches adulthood, it can survive as long as a year without a meal. Thus bedbugs can remain in hiding in vacant apartments and houses, waiting with incredible patience for new tenants to move in, though they may grow lean in the interval. As we have noted, their bodies are flat, especially during periods of starvation. Thus they are able to hide in tiny cracks and crannies, where they are very difficult to detect.

All is not grim in the age-old feud between man and the bedbug that insists on sharing his sheets. In fact, bedbug infestation can have its amusing moments. For example, in England some time ago bedbugs were scattered about in epidemic proportions. During this period ladies who rode the tramcars found the backs of their legs, especially in the regions behind the knee, itching like fury. The gentlemen who occupied the seats beside them appeared to suffer no such discomfort. No doubt they even considered such a reaction some sort of female hysteria. On closer inspection it was discovered that bedbugs had taken up residence in the grooves along the edges of the seats where the more or less unprotected legs of the women were wont to rest. The bedbugs in the interests of survival had turned their nocturnal pattern around to fit the circumstances: by day they arranged themselves in a sociable row to dine on the legs of lady passengers, then by night hid in the tramcar barn in the vehicle of their choice.

In England the bedbug has an odd look-alike, the martin bug, so called because of its habit of residing in the nests of martins. The bugs migrate into homes on occasion, usually through the windows of bedrooms, where their appearance naturally upset fastidious housewives. Authorities report that they are often consulted by distraught homemakers who wish to know how to get rid of the "bedbugs." The martin bug bites, but it has not been demonstrated that it prefers human blood. What really delights it is the blood of martins. Since the English delight in their martins, and since the birds often build their nests in a row under the eaves, martin bugs are likely to be present in large numbers. The English do not like to destroy the martin nests after the birds are gone south, for fear that they will not return the following year, and the martin bugs are likely to get hungry when the birds have flown. A few people are sensitive to their bite, but most are little affected.

In contrast to this look-alike, bedbugs will seek other warm-blooded animals, such as cows, horses, and rates, if human hosts are unavailable. Of course, besides our special type there are species-specific bedbugs. One type of bedbug lives only upon bats, and another prefers chimney swifts. While bedbugs have been indicted as disease carriers, they have never been proved guilty. Still their probing about for a meal and the saliva secretions that accompany their dining can cause uncomfortable, if mild, symptoms. Such symptoms are itching red spots that are usually discovered in the morning as one prepares to rise and begin the day. There are some similarities in the bites of bedbugs, mosquitoes, and fleas, but bedbugs are apt to take their meals in a linear pattern, proceeding from breakfast to lunch to dinner. If one discovers bites in a line, possesses no dog or cat, cannot remember the whine of a mosquito during the night, and is confronted by an unpleasant odor and telltale brownish spots on the sheets, it is time to make a close inspection of the bedding, the mattress, the whole bedroom.

A few individuals are hypersensitive to bedbug bites and exhibit not only marked swelling at the sites but also generalized systemic symptoms as well. There are even a few cases on record of bedbug victims suffering an anaphylactic-shock reaction.

Bedbugs can administer a shock to one's civilized senses. One gentleman retired for the night feeling just fine but woke up before the night was half gone with his face covered with wheals, and his eyes rapidly swelling shut. Cold compresses plus medication relieved the intense itching that accompanied these symptoms, and the wheals disappeared shortly. But his peace of mind was not so easily restored, for his bed was found later to be fully occupied by bedbugs.

One correspondent wrote me from India about an unsettling experience that he had had with bedbugs. He was sleeping in a woven-cane charpoy at a government resthouse when he was awakened by something biting him on the back of his legs, thighs, and back. He moved to a deck chair but soon began wheezing and experiencing breathing difficulties. His face by this time was swollen, especially around the lips. He took several antihistamines that he had with him, and by dawn he had recovered. In his letter he mentioned that he had never had asthma before and that the only allergy he had that he knew about was a penicillin reaction he had suffered some years before.

Bedbugs can be more than a social embarrassment.

BEDBUGS

READER'S GUIDE TO BEDBUGS:

Know the enemy:

Bedbugs are flat and reddish brown in color changing to red when engorged with blood. **(See Plate 28.)**

Treatment of bedbug bites:

It is always prudent to wash any insect bite thoroughly with soap and water. Unless there are symptoms of secondary infection or of a systemic reaction, the only other treatment is to relieve the itching. For instance, calamine lotion may be applied to the bite area. Oral antihistamines may help, but antihistamines should be avoided in lotions or ointments, for the patient may develop a contact dermatitis from them that will put the original bite symptoms in the shade.

How to avoid bedbug infestation and get rid of them once they have moved in:

Cleanliness is the next thing to being bedbug free. Frequent washing of bedding and frequent cleaning of the bedroom will go a long way to discourage bedbugs. If they should move in, let us say, from the vacant apartment upstairs, an insecticide spray is the answer to the problem, with special attention paid to the baseboards, bedstead and frame, and mattress. One of the most effective chemicals is pyrethrum, and it can be applied several times at intervals of one or two weeks. If infestation is heavy, then bedroom walls, upholstered furniture, and the like should also be sprayed.

If the use of insecticides is inadvisable for one reason or another, it is possible to get rid of most, if not all the bedbugs in a room by closing the doors and the windows and turning up the heat to a hundred degrees or more. Several hours of this kind of roasting will usually suffice.

18
The Assassin Bugs

Assassins are secret murderers. The word *assassin*, meaning "a taker of hashish," is derived from that strange eleventh-century Mohammedan organization of killers who believed it their sacred duty to murder anyone who they considered to be an enemy of their semimilitary, fanatical sect. Their leader, known as the Old Man of the Mountain, sent them on their gory forays from an impregnable string of castles in the mountains of Persia. They terrorized their area of the world until they were finally put down in the thirteenth century. These hit men of their time were made maniacal and oblivious to their own hazard by a combination of hashish in the here and now and promises of a paradise in the future complete with dancing girls and gourmet dishes.

What has this to do with bugs? Not a thing really, except that the assassin bugs are the secret murderers of the insect world. Although distantly related to bedbugs, since they too belong to the order Hemiptera, they do not resemble their cousins in the least. With some notable exceptions assassin bugs do not seek out human beings to suck their blood. When they bite us, it is generally in self-defense. Their real pleasure and purpose in life is to prey upon their fellow insects, many of which are clearly our enemies. Thus they are deserving more of our praise than of our censure, although one who has been bitten by an assassin bug may find it hard to praise them: their bite can be painful.

There are about four thousand different species of assassin bugs, and they come in all sizes. One common feature is possessed by all: a powerful beak. With this short but very strong organ they suck the vital fluids out of other insects, and sometimes they suck the blood of mammals, including men. One species, called the Mexican bedbug or big bedbug, slips into houses in the South and West in search of human blood. Not only does it seek our blood but also, along with some near cousins, it transmits a highly fatal disease, called Chagas' disease or, technically, American trypanosomiasis, more popularly known as sleeping sickness.

There are other vectors for sleeping sickness, such as ticks, mites, and mosquitoes, but the species of assassin bugs that transmits the disease most frequently lives cheek by jowl with the victims, hiding in the cracks of flooring and in the walls of flimsy houses. The rats, opossums, and other small animals that are the reservoirs for the disease often live beneath the buildings. The trypanosomes, which cause the disease, are minute parasitic protozoa that invade the blood of many animals. They develop within the insect vector and are passed on when the insect deposits feces on the skin. The contaminated feces are either rubbed into the skin when the host scratches or transmitted to the eyes, nose, or mouth by the fingers. Symptoms of the disease often begin in the eye because it is the area most often contaminated. Eye and face swell in what is known as "the sign of Romana." The victim may be ill for many months with a high fever, anemia, and inflammation of the lymph glands and then die suddenly when the heart is affected. Children are especially afflicted by the acute form of the disease.

Chagas' disease occurs most frequently in Central and South America, but cases have been reported as far north as Texas. The protozoa responsible for the disease have been found in reservoir animals in the Southwest and in some southern states so that the possibility for hazard exists well within our own borders.

Another species of assassin bug, which originated in Europe but somehow got transported to New York, has migrated to the South, where it wanders into homes and occasionally dines on human hosts. Mainly it feeds on the bedbugs some of us have in residence. It is called "the masked hunter" because as a larva it collects dust on the sticky hairs that cover its body, and the dust remains adhered to it for the rest of its life, giving it a strange appearance.

The two species of assassin bug that most interest us here are the kissing bug and the wheel bug, both of which bite. On occasion their bites can inflict local and even systemic reactions in the sensitive.

The kissing bug acquired its rather odd name from its habit of biting its victim on the face. Although its food preferences probably run most to grasshoppers, June bugs, and rats, it deliberately seeks us out, especially while we are asleep. Some varieties apparently consider human beings to be gourmet dining.

There is some confusion of titles among the kissing-bug group of assassins. They go by various names: conenosed bug, Mexican bedbug, China bedbug, Texas bedbug, and bloodsuckers. A number of species are found in the South and Southwest, and one species is predominant on the Pacific Coast. In general they have similar habits and are of a somewhat similar appearance, being flat of body and brown or black in color. Some species, which are found over wide areas of the South and Southwest, have orange markings.

Though they possess wings, kissing bugs are not really fliers. Rather they scurry and scuttle with great speed into cracks and crannies, much as cockroaches do. Because of this and because of their nocturnal habits, they are a rare sight. In warm climates they remain on the prowl all year, but in colder areas they slow down their activities in the winter and bide their time until spring reactivates their urge for blood and biting.

When the kissing bug bites, it extends its long proboscis, in which several hollow stylets are concealed. One of the stylets painlessly penetrates the victim's skin, and the bug settles down to dine. Dining out for this species is a somewhat long-drawn-out affair: in laboratory experiments it was found that it takes as long as eight to twelve minutes for the bug to become engorged. Often as not the kissing bug stands beside its victim to feed rather than climbing aboard. Nor is this disdainful diner satisfied with one bite: often the victim wakes in the morning to find multiple lesions on a face unblemished the night before.

The victim's reaction to kissing-bug bites depends on how many times he has been bitten and how sensitive he is. Researchers have noted four different stages of reaction. Mildly sensitive victims exhibit pimplelike lesions at the bite sites that are usually a little more marked than other insect bites, or small blisterlike vesicles may show up in a group at one bite site without a central lesion. A more sensitive victim may find large wheals on his face the morning after with a good deal of contiguous swelling. In a severe reaction there may be purplish nodules or blisterlike lesions on the hands and feet as well as the face. Individuals who have been bitten previously by kissing bugs tend to have more severe reactions than do those encountering the bug for the first time. Sensitization takes place, and the person becomes allergic to kissing bugs after an initial attack. But that is not the whole story. One researcher, bravely exposed himself repeatedly to a kissing bug's appetite, discovered that his reaction became increasingly severe the more he was bitten but that finally he developed a certain immunity, for his reactions began gradually to diminish in intensity.

Physicians have recorded various symptoms following kissing-bug bites: itching at the bite site, generalized itching over the entire body, widespread hives, fainting, nausea and vomiting, swollen eyes, breathing difficulties, and difficulty in swallowing and speaking because of swelling in the mouth and throat. A number of anaphylactic shock reactions have also been recorded.

The following case demonstrates the damage a kissing bug can do. A woman patient woke at dawn one day to find her whole body itching. Feeling nauseated, she rose to go to the bathroom, but felt so faint that she had to lie down on the floor. Unable to rise and feeling deathly ill, she vomited where she lay. By the time she arrived in a hospital emergency room, she had returned to normal, but her face was swollen, and she suffered from widespread hives. She reported that at the height of her illness she had felt a tightness in her throat, a sense of constriction, a symptom characteristic of a generalized systemic reaction.

As I was preparing this book, a colleague sent me a newspaper clipping recording the death of a man bitten by a kissing bug. The unfortunate man, who was in his forties, had suffered a fatal systemic reaction. It was the first documented case of such a fatality in California. According to the dead man's family he had been bitten several times before by this kind of bug and had suffered allergic reactions. Because of his somewhat unusual response he had collected data on the bug, becoming interested in his own particular nemesis.

As I mentioned earlier, the odd thing is that, when the kissing bug is actually biting, there is no pain. People sleep through the bite and the bloodsucking to wake to the results the next morning. It must be a somewhat puzzling experience, and naturally the horrifying thought of bedbugs may first come to mind. However, as we have noted, bedbugs commonly bite in a linear pattern—one, two, three. They also emit a characteristicaly pungent odor and leave reddish-brown tracks on the sheets. Spiders can inflict bites similar to those of the kissing bug, but they usually bite only once. Kissing-bug bites tend to be multiple and grouped.

The second assassin bug common to our land that causes a bit of human misery is the wheel bug, so named because of the odd and distinctive feature on the top of the front part of its body. This is a sort of ridged crest strongly resembling part of a cogged wheel. The wheel bug makes its home throughout most of the United States, from south of New York all the way west to Texas and New Mexico. It likes to dwell under rocks and debris. Gray in color, the wheel bug is a fairly large insect. The female may be 1 or 1¼ inches in size, which makes her rather formidable in contrast to the rest of the insect world. Like its other assassin cousins the wheel bug possesses a strong, jointed, beaklike proboscis. It has long, slender antennae and front legs that resemble those of a praying mantis. Its legs are long and strong, ideally suited to grasp its prey.

Human beings make contact with the wheel bug's painful bite when we disturb it in its crannies or when it is attracted to our porches by lights at night or when a heavy rain drives it to seek shelter in our homes. The bugs do not particularly care for our blood, but they dislike being handled roughly. Unfortunately, their salivary secretions are toxic, for they are designed to kill their insect prey. When injected into human beings, the secretions produce reactions that vary from a temporary local lesion, which hurts but presents no real problem, to widespread benign growths on the skin somewhat resembling warts. Generally it is a question of severe pain and a lesion that persists for only a few hours.

One physician wrote to me about two of his patients who encountered the assassins. The first was a teenage boy who ran afoul of a conenosed bug, whose identity is not known, while he was loading trash cans. The pain of the bite and the resulting redness lasted less than half an hour. The second case was that of a little girl, who acquired a wheel bug in her shoe and sustained a very painful bite on the foot. Both the pain and the lesion were cleared up within fifteen to twenty minutes. The physician went on to say that neither patient required medication and he was not informed about any delayed reaction and so could assume that was all there was to both cases. Apparently we have little to fear from the wheel bug, although I myself would go out of my way to avoid even the temporary discomfort of its bite.

There is one odd feature to the wheel bug's attack that has been mentioned by some of its victims: the bite area becomes warmer than surrounding tissue and may remain that way for many months, long after the memory of the pain that the wheel bug caused has vanished. One patient, who was bitten on the finger, reported that a year later the finger felt warmer than the rest of his hand.

All in all, the assassins are far more of a threat to their fellow insects than they are to us but like the Old Man of the Mountain, they lurk unpleasantly in hidden places. They are beneficial because they do away with a good many insect pests, but they are also potentially harmful as disease vectors.

READER'S GUIDE TO ASSASSIN BUGS:

Know the enemy:

- The kissing bug is flat and brown or black in color. Some species flaunt orange markings. **(See Plate 29.)**
- The wheel bug is mouse gray in color and may be as large as 1 or 1¼ inches. It has a distinctive crest over the head that looks like part of a cog or a geared wheel. **(See Plate 30.)**

What to do if bitten by an assassin bug:

Treatment—if any is needed, and often it is not—is much the same as for any other insect bite. The important thing is to wash the bite area well with soap and water and apply an antiseptic. Mild sedatives may help if pain is severe. Of course, if signs of an infection or of a systemic reaction develop, a physician should be consulted at once, for antibiotics or other medications may be necessary.

How to avoid being bitten by an assassin bug:

It is impossible to guard against accidental collision with an assassin bug, but, steps can be taken to minimize the chances of an encounter. Since assassin bugs frequent the burrows of rodents, keeping the home area free of trash piles, undisturbed stacks of lumber, and the like will go a long way in controlling assassin populations. Care should be taken not to bring the bugs into the house on firewood, laundry, and the like. Keeping the bedroom especially clean will help keep the kissing bug at bay. Finally, it is well to wear gloves and to look first before handling such things as logs, lumber, and trash.

19

Beetles: Of Beauty and Blisters

We have dealt thoroughly with the insects that most frequently pose health problems for human beings, but there are always surprises in life. There is always an aberrant villain lurking about to catch us unawares. Not many people run afoul of beetles, for instance, but the few who do encounter certain beetle species have cause to regret the chance acquaintance.

There are well over 200,000 different species of beetles, which belong to the order Coleoptera. Some of them are beautiful. Some tiger-beetle species, for example, come in purple, green, blue, scarlet, and orange. The metallic wood-boring beetles are often brillantly colored and iridescent, although in some species the color shows only when they are in flight. At rest on the tree trunk that they are busy boring, they appear much like a lump of bark. Even that pest the Japanese beetle is a thing of beauty, if one can be objective about it.

Beetles have been remarkably successful in the battle for survival. There are some odd-looking characters among them, and some with very odd habits. There is, for instance, the rhinoceros dung beetle, which is aptly named since it looks exactly like a miniature rhinoceros, complete with horn. One type of click beetle has spots that look for all the world like giant eyes. The click beetle has provided hours of amusement for many a youngster. Placed on its back, it may wave its legs feebly for about a minute as though trying desperately to right itself. Then suddenly it will snap its hinged body several inches into the air and, chance willing, land right side up. Since chance and children are fickle, it will probably promptly end up on its back again.

Tumblebugs, or dung beetles, bury enormous amounts of manure in the soil, much to the benefit of the soil and human sanitation. Some of them are ball rollers, forming the manure into a ball, which they push to wherever they have chosen to dine. Then they bury both dung and themselves to eat in leisure. When the cupboard is bare, they surface to go after another bit of manure. Often several beetles work together to secure a ball and move it to their hideout. It is quite a sight to see one or two beetles no more than an inch long pushing a ball of manure the size of a baseball along the ground. They accomplish this trick by backing along, pushing at the ball with their hind legs. Dung beetles account for a good deal of manure going underground to enrich the soil. One researcher reported that one dung beetle buried sixty cubic inches of the stuff in one night.

There are carrion beetles, including the burying beetle, which are capable of burying the carcass of a small animal. They undermine the dirt beneath the carcass until it sinks into the disturbed soil. Thus they give the dead decent burial and fill their own larder at the same time.

Then, of course, there are the fireflies. This beetle has been a source of wonder down through the centuries, but only recently have we tried to penetrate the mystery of the firefly's "cold" light. So far our intelligence has not succeeded in producing light nearly as efficiently with as great a saving in energy as it does. Nor do we know just how this particular beetle achieves the feat; it is still an entrancing mystery. We do know what substances are involved: luciferin, luciferase, and adenosine triphosphate. When the first two chemicals come into contact with the third—producing a compound that exists in all living cells—light is made by the firefly. If fireflies, to their misfortune, are ground up, the resulting product will continue to glow, but if the luciferase is destroyed, the light vanishes. One of the ways that the Viking vehicle on Mars tested for the presence of life was to add these chemicals, luciferin and luciferase, to a scoop of soil. Presumably, if there was life as we know it in the soil, there would be a glow that could be registered on sensitive instruments, and the result could be sent back to earth. In the same manner bacteria in water and air can be readily detected. Since luciferin has been synthesized in the laboratory, the need to grind up harmless fireflies has diminished.

The very existence of fireflies has been threatened in recent decades. Not only have they been called upon to give their all for science, but pollution has all but wiped them out in some places in the world. The Japanese, who traditionally have an eye for beauty, became so concerned about their technological decimation of the lightening bug that they appropriated money to restore the firefly to their land. It is a terrible thought that there may be children in the future who will never have the opportunity to chase after the blinking beetle on a summer's evening. I would have hated to miss that.

Some strange things about fireflies seem more fiction than fact. Yet competent, objective observers have noticed them. For instance, in some areas, particularly in South America, it has been observed that all the fireflies on one side of a river winked in unison while the fireflies on the opposite bank winked in unison on a different beat. The fireflies on, say, the left bank would be answered seconds later by the fireflies on the right bank, and on ad infinitum. How do they synchronize such a business? Apparently nobody knows, although various theories have been suggested, ranging from the idea that the flashs are almost instantaneous responses to the hypothesis that an internal pacemaker regulates the rhythm of the group. We know that the flashes are mating signals to bring boy and girl fireflies together, but, strangely enough, there are nonluminous firefly species that are at least as numerous as their lit-up cousins. Somehow or other they manage to propagate their kind without the need for lanterns. Even stranger, it is said that frogs, who are apparently very fond of eating fireflies, glow around the stomach region if they ingest enough of this special treat. A crew of lit-up frogs sitting on lily pads about a pond could be quite a sight.

All in all, the firefly is a thing of beauty. Bless it and keep it for our children and for the childlike wonder that we should maintain in our hearts all our days. And the firefly is friendly: it does us no harm.

So it is also with the ladybug, or, more technically, the lady beetle. Would that we had more friends like them in the insect world. The lady bug is death to aphids and scale insects that infest our gardens and flower beds. One patient researcher tallied the take of a lady beetle and found that in the larval stage alone a single lady beetle consumed 90 aphids and 3,000 scale insects. Such a prodigious appetite accompanies the lady beetle into adulthood. So we can imagine what the eventual tally would be. Small wonder that this little predator is a collector's item packaged and advertised in seed catalogs as a must for the gardener. In California, for instance, lady beetles gather in colonies to overwinter. They are tenderly garnered and sold to citrus growers. Without the lady beetle our gardens would be overrun, or we would have to drown them with insecticides. She and the praying mantis are insects to be cherished.

Alas, the bean beetle belongs in the same, otherwise eminently respectable family, and anyone who mistakes the bean beetle for a friend is likely to lose his beans. They are voracious, and once they attack, a bean plant succumbs rapidly. It seems a low blow of nature to have included this bean destroyer in the lady-beetle family. Still, its existence is no excuse for a gentleman, young or old, to step upon a ladybug. Which is probably why children still chant the old ditty:

> Ladybug, ladybug,
> Fly away home.
> Your house is on fire,
> Your children are gone,
> All except Ann,
> Who hid under the pudding pan.

That is the version that I remember. I expect there are dozens of others.

Thus beetles can be helpful as well as harmful to humans. Tiger beetles consume quantities of insects that we rate as pests. Ground beetles, of which there are more than 20,000 species, do away with caterpillars and other pests, including snails, which is all very well as long as you are not raising snails for the gourmet's table. Water beetles of one type or another slaughter a good many pests. Some of their species are so wolfish that they also do away with fish much larger than themselves. How they manage such a feat is interesting, if ghoulish. As larvae they have long, curving mouthparts with hollow canals in the centers. When they get a hold on a small fish, they hang on grimly and pump digestive substances into the victim. Slowly but surely, the fish's tissues are liquefied and consumed until there is nothing left but an empty shell. Obviously, neither the fish farmer nor the dedicated fisherman is going to look upon this kind of thing calmly.

The beetles that we are most concerned about in this book are the blister beetle and its cousin the oil beetle. Nature has provided these beetles with a particularly chancy means of survival. The female lays between two thousand and ten thousand eggs in or on the ground, then goes about her business with no thought of providing a larder for her offspring. When they hatch, it is up to the larvae to find their host, which is either locust eggs or the nests of solitary bees, who do provide for their progeny. Those larvae for whom locust eggs are the proper host set off on a ground search. Those who must end up in a solitary-bee nest in order to survive climb up into flowers and wait. If they mistakenly latch on to a fly or a honeybee, their doom is sealed. When they do find the species of host that nature has chosen for them it must be a female solitary bee. Now and again a larva that has latched onto the wrong sex of the proper host will be lucky enough to be able to transfer to the female during mating, but the odds must surely be against this change in flight. In fact, the odds are so heavily against the thousands of hatched larvae that only a few manage to catch a ride with the right lady bee. When they do succeed, they slip into the egg cell that she has prepared and provisioned. Sealed in with the bee egg, the beetle larva quickly consumes the egg, then turns at its leisure to the pollen and the nectar intended for its victim. Dining thus in peace and quiet, it goes through its various molting stages and emerges eventually as a pupa one step from adulthood.

These beetles are a hazard for us, though, because they exude a powerful substance, cantharidin, when disturbed. Cantharidin is so powerful that a tiny drop can burn like fire and raise a large blister on human skin. In past centuries, when blistering and bleeding were the two great cures, cantharidin was liberally employed by physicians for the former treatment. It also had a great popularity as an aphrodisiac—the Spanish fly—but it proved to be somewhat hazardous. It also did not live up to expectations: it simply did not work.

The majority of our blister beetles reside in the western half of the United States and are most active during the height of summer. They range in size from a quarter inch to an inch and have a characteristic leathery look. Eastern varieties are generally deep purple in color; western varieties, commonly ash-colored.

Since blister beetles fly about at night and are attracted to lights, their victims are likely to be people standing around under a street light waiting for a bus, sitting in a porch swing with a light above their heads, or enjoying a stand-up cocktail party in the garden under colorful Japanese lanters. If the blister beetle is allowed to walk unhampered down your arm or leg, it will do you no harm. But when you try to brush it off, or if it feels the pressure of an article of clothing, ouch!

When pressure is exerted on the beetle, it exudes fluid from its knee joints, genital region, and other areas of its body. The secretion usually causes a slight tingling initially. A slight rash may appear. About eight to ten hours later a large blister will have formed. Sometimes there is only a single blister, but often they are multiple, for the skin reacts wherever the cantharidin has been distributed by the leaking beetle. If the blisters are not ruptured, they will usually be reabsorbed within a few days. If they are ruptured, the skin will flake, and except for a mild reddening of the area, all signs will vanish in a week or so. In general, the attack of the blister beetle is a mild business although temporarily somewhat disfiguring. On occasion, however, cantharidin can do more than blister the skin. It has a penetrating action, and it can irritate the kidneys. If ingested, it can cause nausea, diarrhea, vomiting, and painful abdominal cramps.

We can readily imagine the dismay of the woman who wore an off-the-shoulder dress at the garden party from whose un-blemished skin a gallant gentleman knocked off a blister bee-tle. The gentleman was a bit awkward in this maneuver, and the lady's shoulders and arms were quite a mess. Victims often show the results of a blister beetle's meanderings over their skin. Feet, ankles, wrists, neck, and even the soles of the feet are the areas most frequently affected. Wherever the skin is most exposed is usually the site of the attack. The contrary was reported a good many years ago when the English colony in the Sudan suffered an epidemic of blister-beetle attacks while the natives were unaffected. The English suffered doubtless because they wore too many clothes, while the na-tives went about in a state of undress. The blister beetles crawled up unnoticed under the English clothing and exuded as they felt the pressure of all that civilized covering. It should also be noted that some species of blister beetle are fond of such crops as potatoes, tomatoes, beans, corn, and fruit and thus pose a problem for farm workers.

While blister-beetle blisters are unsightly, they are usually temporary and pose no great problem for human beings. I do not know of any case of systemic reaction following a blister beetle's release of cantharidin on the skin. Physicians may have some difficulty in diagnosis if the patient does not re-member anything crawling over his skin, but good indica-tions of blister-beetle attack are that the blisters, if there are more than one, are all in the same stage of development and there is no accompanying rash around them. The slight initial reddening vanishes by the time the blisters appear in their full glory.

I have not heard that the blister beetle transmits disease,

even indirectly. All in all, we cannot really work up a very blistering indictment of this beetle. Nevertheless, it is best avoided.

READER'S GUIDE TO BLISTER BEETLES:

Know the enemy:

The blister beetle ranges in size from ¼ inch to 1 inch. It is somewhat soft of body and has a rather broad head and narrow neck. Blister beetles in the eastern United States are purplish in color. Those of the West are commonly ash gray. **(See Plate 31.)**

Treatment for blisters resulting from the beetle's discharge of cantharidin on the skin:

Small lesions should be protected by Band-Aids or bandages until they reabsorb. A mild antiseptic ointment can be applied to the area as a precautionary measure, but a thorough soap-and-water wash is as good as anything. Large blisters, especially those occurring on the feet, should be seen by a physician. He will probably trim off the blister, drain it, and apply antiseptics and bandages. If the feet are blistered, walking should be avoided as much as possible.

20

Caterpillars
and Other Oddities

About three centuries before Christ a Chinese philosopher, Chuang Tzu, said, "I do not know whether I was then a man dreaming I was a butterfly, or whether I am now a butterfly dreaming I am a man." No philosopher that I know of has ever dreamed that he was a caterpillar, and the reason, I think, is obvious: who would want to be a creepy, crawly thing if he could dream of assuming the colors of the rainbow and of flitting freely across the sunlit meadows of the world. It is sad that before there can be a butterfly there must first be a soft-bodied, sluggish creature twice cursed for its destructiveness to the crops, trees, and flowers so cherished by human beings. Caterpillars are the larvae of the butterflies and moths that make up the order Lepidoptera, a large and often incredibly beautiful group of insects. While one may think twice about destroying a gorgeous creature of many colors, it is rare that one hesitates when confronted by an inch-long, greenish, wormlike beast busily chewing on a prized cabbage plant. It takes some doing for a caterpillar ever to metamorphose into a butterfly or its draber cousin the moth.

The word *caterpillar* derives from the Latin for "hairy cat." Certainly a good many caterpillars are hairy, and I suppose some of them have a catlike appearance. What caterpillars do best is eat, eat, eat, as most of us who garden are ruefully aware. In essence the caterpillar is a mobile mouth, its mouth-parts are efficiently engineered as perfect plant grinders. Its eyes, six in a curving row on each side of its prominent head, apparently function just well enough for it to distinguish vertical stems and tree trunks on which to forage for food. The first three segments are the thorax, and the rest are the abdomen. Each thorax segment bears a pair of legs that will eventually be a pair of legs on the mature insect. The abdomen segments also supply the caterpillar with legs, five pairs in all, but these disappear in the final stages of molting. Instead of feet, these legs end in tiny hooks, the better to hold the caterpillar to a stem or leaf or whatever.

The caterpillar possesses one strange feature, a spinneret located on the lower lip. Its life literally hangs by a thread, for wherever the caterpillar goes, whatever it does, it spins out a tiny thread along the way. As the spinneret lays down this sticky thread, the minute feet grip it, and in this way the caterpillar can maneuver over all sorts of steep and slick surfaces. If it falls, the thread continues to spin a bit until the caterpillar can get a grip and climb back up to resume its journey along the path that it lays down for itself. Frequently, when about to be gulped down by a bird, a caterpillar deliberately falls down its thread, leaving a startled bird behind. For all its sharpsightedness the bird often does not spot the insect dangling a few feet below.

Some caterpillars have nests, to which they return each night along the thread that they spin by day. Others that bore into wood line the resulting hole with their silk, transforming an ordinary hole into a luxurious home. And, of course, when the time comes to molt, members of some species knit themselves a snug silk cocoon. Some species that live a kind of primitive communal life spin a tent nest, in which they all crowd during the night and when inclement weather makes forays for food uncomfortable or downright hazardous for such cold-blooded beasts. The way they construct their tent is intriguing: after consuming a great amount of food, the caterpillars seek a warm, sunny spot to digest it. As they cluster together, they spin their threads, and as they move about, they gradually form mats of silk among branches of a bush or tree. As the tent forms, the caterpillars move about behind its sheltering walls, creating an ever-larger tent and even compartments within the tent.

When it comes to self-defense, caterpillars are a pretty helpless lot. Some of them are fortunate enough to be clothed in protective coloring of sorts, a pattern of fairly good camouflage that blends with the light and shadow of foliage. Others possess frightening-looking horns that scare would-be predators away. Others can lash their "tails" to appear a good deal more formidable than they are. Some even have special organs that they can pop out of their bodies when they are attacked, giving off unpleasant odors or giving the caterpillars themselves a nasty flavor. This may not help the caterpillar that is scooped up by, say, a bird, and then is spat out in a damaged state, but it helps the particular species.

The caterpillars that we are concerned with here are those that contain hollow spines or hairs that secrete a poison when the caterpillar is handled. These are called urticating caterpillars. There are several species capable of damaging the human hide and of inflicting a painful sting. Worse still, systemic reactions may occur, and sometimes they can be severe, even fatal.

One species of urticating caterpillar is the larva of the brown-tail moth of New England. When handled, it will leave tiny blisters along the skin wherever it has touched. The adult moth is also capable of causing a dermatitis on contact. If the hairs of the caterpillar get into the eyes, they can cause quite a bit of difficulty, and when the hairs are inhaled or ingested, they can cause serious illness on occasion. Research has shown that toxins in the hairs cause changes in red blood cells, transforming them from their normal round shape into shrunken, knobbed corpuscles and, at the same time, breaking up their normal grouping. Therefore, be warned: do not handle a nearly black caterpillar with brown hairs and a row of white tufts on each of its sides.

Caterpillars and Other Oddities

If you live in Arizona, New Mexico, or the desert regions of California, do not handle the caterpillar of the paloverde buck moth. It is most often found on or in the vicinity of paloverde trees. About 1½ inches long, it is pale greenish-gray with rows of dark hairs springing out from a common axis and with a brown head. This caterpillar can cause an intense pain, reddening and itching at the point of contact, and subsequent blistering. There are no reports of systemic reactions to this particular species, although again uncomfortable eye involvement can occur when the hairs float or are rubbed into the eye.

In the South we have to contend with the saddleback caterpillar, commonly called the packsaddle caterpillar because of a saddlelike appearance. Some people call it the cotton worm since it appears to be most frequently encountered by cotton pickers in the fields. Green, with oval brown dots, it has hairs of a lighter color and seems to possess a head at both ends, although one head is really all nature has provided. It can sting, and one physician has reported a case in which the patient suffered an anaphylactic reaction to its toxin.

It is the puss caterpillar, however, that most often causes harm (although it must be said that victims of caterpillars of any stripe are rare). The puss caterpillar goes by a number of labels: possum bug, woolly worm, Italian asp. There are probably others, and none too flattering, for, by whatever label, this larva of the flannel moth can hurt. The caterpillars frequent gardens, shade trees, and ornamental shrubs in the southern states, where they are numerous.

The puss is shaped like a teardrop and possesses a pointed tail. It varies in length from ½ inch to 1½ inches. Its hairs are tan, darkish gray, and cream in color, and because of this variation of color, the puss is hard to detect on the branch or trunk of a tree. When threatened, they rear up, inflate their heads, and lash their tails, maneuvers guaranteed to make all but the lion-hearted back off.

The puss manufactures a distinctive poison, which it loads in hollow spines located among its long hairs. This toxic substance remains in the spines even after the puss is dead, so a puss carcass should be handled with as much care as a live one, if it must be handled at all.

The puss's sting is painful, far more so than one would think from the resulting lesion. The pain is rhythmic, coming and going like the beat of a drum. It follows almost at once after contact with the puss so that there is no doubt about its cause. The lesion itself exhibits swelling and itching. If a leg or an arm is involved, frequently there is also pain under the arm or in the groin area. Numbness can occur, and the victim is often anxious and restless. The wound region becomes splotched with a red, ridged rash, which may extend over a large area. The whole can itch severely. This syndrome of pain, itching, and lesion may last anywhere from a few hours to a few days.

As a more serious consequence, contact with the puss caterpillar frequently produces systemic symptoms that can be acute. Nausea, fever, and muscle cramps have all been reported. Some patients have developed shock symptoms of rapid heartbeat, widespread itching over the body, and convulsions. Involvement of the lymph glands is also common.

For example, on physician reported on a young woman who stepped barefoot on a puss caterpillar. She felt an instantaneous burning sensation in her foot. Within minutes she was suffering symptoms of shock with respiratory distress. She complained of shooting pains in her leg and groin. When she arrived at the hospital, her blood pressure had fallen, and her pulse was slow. Treatment relieved pain and shock symptoms, although her foot and leg felt numb for several days.

The physician has no difficulty in diagnosing a patient's contact with a puss, for the caterpillar leaves a characteristic gridlike mark, a parallel track of puncture marks surrounded by a white, thickened area. Sometimes the puss leaves a perfect picture of itself in outline on the skin. This distinctive track and the shooting pains that follow the initial itching of the wound area within minutes clearly mark the culprit.

Children especially can have a hard time with the puss caterpillar. About fifty years ago these caterpillars became so numerous in San Antonio, Texas, that the schools had to be closed because many youngsters were stung in or around them. Florida has periodic infestations during which children, born curious, often get stung.

Like other caterpillars, and, for that matter, adult moths and other insects, the puss can cause problems even if it does not sting. The poisonous hairs may cause pulmonary irritation if they are inhaled. They may be the cause, it is conjectured, of sudden and mysterious cases of bronchitis and asthma. The hairs can also get into the eyes to cause irritation. As we shall see in the next chapter, some insects can be a hazard to humans long after they have gone to insect Valhalla.

One strange case of moth attack occurred a number of years ago in the Norwegian crew of a tanker when the ship was well out to sea. Almost every man aboard suddenly developed an intense itch and a rash. The ship radioed for medical advice, saying that the crew had come down with the Caripito Itch, a condition that the sailors were familiar with and that seemed to follow visits to the port of Caripito, Venezuela. In fact, port authorities there had routinely warned sailors against the moth. When the short hairs of the moth's wings or abdomen come into contact with human skin, they can cause swelling, rash, itching, and pimples. Since medical stores on a tanker are somewhat limited, medical advice consisted of the use of ephedrine and a washing with a weak solution of ammonia. The latter was ordinary cleaning ammonia. After a couple of days of such treatment the tanker's captain radioed that his men were much improved. He later informed authorities that he knew of other ships' crews who had been similarly affected in the past.

Sometimes insects appear to go berserk. They seem to be abruptly derailed, leaving their natural state, or at least what we humans are pleased to consider their natural state, to take on new roles. For instance, thrips, which are tiny sapsucking insects, occasionally forsake their diet of plant juices to take after humans. One observer working in an onion patch noticed that onion thrips abandoned their traditional fare to give him a going-over. As he worked he suddenly felt mild pricks on his arms, face, and neck and noticed that little pinkish dots were turning up on his skin. Being of a scientific bent, he peered more closely and calmly noted that thrip larvae were the hungriest and that, as they fed upon him, they turned a reddish color. Others have reported that grass and grain winged thrips are likely to migrate when their specific food supply dries up or is harvested. On their way to new fields of plenty they are likely to feed on any human beings that they encounter.

We do not think of grasshoppers as much of a threat. In truth, they are not except to our crops and the like. But there is always an exception to upset a premise, as the following case illustrates:

> For two autumns running a young teenage boy suffered from widespread hives and edema, or swelling, of his face and hands. The symptoms generally followed football practice. They were bad enough to send him to his physician. Both patient and his mother thought either grasshoppers in the football field or praying mantises might have something to do with his problem. Since there was no family or patient history of allergy, and since grasshoppers have not been considered much of an allergy hazard, this seemed farfetched, but when the young man was skin-tested with grasshopper extract, he turned out to be very sensitive indeed. Desensitization was begun, and by the time football season rolled around again, he was able to enjoy being flung upon the grass without an itch or a rash. As far as his attending physician knew at the time he reported this case, the boy had gone through three football seasons without a recurrence of symptoms.

I do not know what such a case report will do for that perennial old favorite among children's stories, "The Grasshopper and the Ant." I suppose it will add a smidgeon of anxiety to the notion that grasshoppers are merry, if lazy and inclined to fritter their days away. Still, when all is said and done, allergy to grasshoppers has to be rare.

Now we must turn our attention to the rather horrifying notion that the air we breathe, the food that we eat, the water that we drink is loaded with the living and decayed remains, the hairs, the feces, and the general debris of the insect world, and that all this insect garbage presents a health hazard for some of us.

READER'S GUIDE TO CATERPILLARS AND THRIPS:

Know the enemy:

Puss caterpillar:
The puss caterpillar is shaped like a teardrop with a pointed tail. It is tan, darkish gray, and cream in color and ranges anywhere from ½ to 1½ inches in length. **(See Plate 32.)**

Thrip:
The thrip is tiny, so small that it can pass through ordinary screening. It is long and slender without wings, or with very narrow wings.

What to do if stung by a puss caterpillar:

Home treatment:
Apply Scotch tape or adhesive tape over the lesion to remove any broken-off spines that may be embedded in the skin. In mild cases an antihistamine may help to relieve pain. Ice cubes or ammonia applied to the sting area may also help relive pain. Severe reactions should be seen by a physician at once. Ointments or lotions applied to the sting site are not much help.

What to do if stung by other caterpillar species:

Wash the area well with soap and water. Apply a mild antiseptic ointment, preferably in a petrolatum base.

What to do if attacked by thrips or grasshoppers:

Wash the resulting rash or termatitis with soap and water. Consult a physician if systemic symptoms or infection results.

How to avoid the attentions of caterpillars:

Keep the home area clean of debris, especially around flower beds and trees. Wear gloves and other appropriate clothing when working in infested areas (for the puss caterpillar, that is states south of Virginia) to avoid accidental contact. Insecticides may have to be sprayed over large areas of infestation.

21
Insects Inhaled and Ingested

Insect stings and bites are not the only way that bugs, beetles, and bees pose a health hazard for humans. When we were school children, we were told that we should keep food covered lest the fly track filth and germs upon it. A certain fastidiousness, kept the teacher at least during my school days, from referring to cockroaches in the same vein. It was a well-kept secret that roaches would not only track filth over my food but that also vomit and excrete into it. Maybe it was just as well that I never knew such things in my tender years. Childhood's nightmares can be unpleasant enough.

Nor did I learn in school that, when insects of some species depart this life, they leave their carcasses, often dismembered, not only in my food but also in the air that I must breathe. Yes, to be altogether truthful, I am glad I grew up in ignorance. Childhood appetites should remain as undisturbed as possible.

We have already taken a horrified look at dust mites within the home. Insect debris does not stop at our front doors either: shed scales and hairs join particles of wings and bodies, abandoned cocoons and exoskeletons, feces, and secretions, to ride the air currents around us. Naturally, the part of the body most affected by an allergic reaction to these particles is the respiratory system—the lungs, the bronchi, and the nose. Generally symptoms are seasonal, since the insects start each warm period of the year in smallish numbers, then build rapidly to huge populations. Thus the insects that swarm in profusion cause the most damage. Some species, such as mayflies and caddis flies, fill the air with adults within a very short time span. They dance their day or so of maturity, then mate and die, leaving their bodies to disintegrate and blow upon the wind. Thus a great wealth of dead animal matter accompanies the air into our noses and lungs.

Oddly enough, those who are sensitive to this debris react with symptoms of allergy—usually hay-fever symptoms or asthma—to the debris of either the class Insecta or the class Arachnida without a crossover of sensitivity. Thus, if you are sensitive to the debris of cockroaches, you will probably not be bothered by the house-dust mite, and vice versa. Laboratory studies suggest that, if you are allergic to insects within an order of one class, you will probably cross-react to some degree to all members of that order. Studies have indicated that the larvae and pupae of insects contain allergenic substances akin to those found within the adult forms. Dead or alive, insects seem determined to cause us trouble. Studies and surveys indicate that allergic reactions to inhaled insect debris are rather common. These allergies have been pinpointed in one study as more prevalent in the Appalachian mountain region than along the East Coast or in the Midde West. Men seem to suffer from them more frequently than do women, perhaps because their occupations take them outdoors more often.

It is not fully known which substances in insect debris are the cause of allergy symptoms, but it is thought that the protein content of insect chitin (the hard, horny substance of the insect's exterior), a similar protein in insect silk, and the protein of arthropodin (a substance found in the limbs of spiders, ticks, and the like) are the substances most likely to do damage to the allergic individual's respiratory system. Insect hairs, which are often so profuse in the air that they can be observed, may irritate the respiratory tract, and the hairs of some insects, such as the puss caterpillar, contain toxic substances that are still viable after they are separated from the insect itself.

A correlation between insect-inhalant allergy and three insect types has been well documented: mayflies, caddis flies, and house-dust mites. The insects in question swarm in great numbers, usually within limited time spans. The relationship with allergy is clear because a good many patients turn up with symptoms of hay fever and asthma during the periods when the insects swarm and then are skin-tested and diagnosed as allergic to those particular insects.

Medical attention first focused on the mayfly as a culprit. It was noticed that its annual swarming coincided with a good deal of temporary respiratory discomfort that was regional in character. In late spring or early summer mayflies appear in huge clouds along lake shores and riverbanks in various parts of the world, probably nowhere more than in the Great Lakes area of the United States. As a larva the mayfly dwells in the water and is entirely aquatic, obtaining oxygen by means of a kind of gill structure. Its brief foray into the air is the last day of its life. The very name of the order to which it belongs, Ephemeroptera, derives from the Greek for "lasting but a day."

Called variously shad flies, willow flies, day flies, lake flies, eel flies, and cob flies, mayflies spend from one to four years as larvae and nymphs in the water, feeding on plant tissue and readying themselves for their one great day, or hour as the case may be. Some mayfly species emerge from the water, go through their final molt to adulthood, mate, and die all within the space of an hour or two.

Once mature, the mayfly does not eat again. Nor does it crawl or walk. It only flies, and it joins its brethren and sistern to fly in dancing swarms. In late afternoon or early evening the swarms, consisting of hundreds or thousands of the small insects, rise and fall over lake shores and riverbanks. When a male and a female meet, it is love on first flight. They take off together to ensure that mayflies will return for their day in the future. Then the female, chockablock with eggs, flies over water to scatter them, although in some species she lays them en masse in a suitable place. Once the last egg is laid, she herself falls to the water's surface and drifts off to insect Valhalla. The females of some species lay their eggs under water beneath a stone. They simply dive down with their load and never come up, presumably finding their way to Valhalla on underwater currents.

In the meantime in the air, as the dancing swarms run out of time, their bodies and the skins of their final molts fall in such numbers to earth that they litter the shores of lakes and ponds and may put out campfires. Car windshields in the area become so spattered that driving is difficult. Sidewalks and porches of lake-shore towns must be swept daily, for the accumulated carcasses can reach a depth of several inches and can make footing mighty slippery. Off-water breezes often blow the swarms some distance inland to share the burden of windrows of mayfly bodies.

Such brief lives may seem sad to us, but for some of us there is additional cause for regret. A reasonably large number of people who dwell where mayflies dance and shower their debris toward earth come down with a sensonal hay fever and, sometimes, serious asthma.

Caddis flies follow a somewhat similar pattern of life. They too live in water as larvae and come to the surface only for their final molt to maturity. The adults then also form dense clouds that hover in the air. They are seldom seen by day, for they hide in brush and grass near water and come out to fly at night. Since they are drawn to lights, we become aware of their existence then. They often slip into our homes when porch lights and lighted windows bring them into the vicinity.

Caddis flies are closely related to moths, though their lives until adulthood are totally unlike that of their moth cousins. From the point of view of oddity, the larva stage is the most interesting. Many of the three thousand different species build strange cases into which part of their body fits. Hooks at their posterior ends keep them within the cases, although their heads and long legs may extend out of the opening in front. What is truly remarkable is that some species weave sand particles, pebbles, even twigs into the sticky silk of the cases. Some even use twigs to construct a little wood-and-silk shanty. Bubbles of air trapped within the case lighten the load for the larva so that it can flip about in the water on its never-ending search for food. Some species of caddis fly build nets or traps; they then depend upon the currents to fill these larders.

When the time to pupate arrives, the larva seals itself in its case, leaving only enough of an opening for water to circulate around it, since this is its source of oxygen. When it is time to emerge, it cuts itself free, rises swiftly to the surface and splits, and the adult caddis fly is there to shake out its wings and be up and away before those precious wings can get wet.

Like the mayfly the caddis fly lives not to eat and make merry but to love and to die. And it is this end to their tale that causes some of us to sneeze and wheeze, for again, as with the mayfly, the caddis fly strews its debris and its carcasses into the air, over food we eat, into water we drink.

Even aphids—those tiny, defenseless honey pots of the ant kingdom—dry up at the end of their life cycle to join the general insect garbage that is scattered throughout the environment. Because aphids are so plentiful, they also are a force to be reckoned with when it comes to allergy of the respiratory system.

Does the reader doubt that there is so much insect debris floating about? Note the following: About thirty years ago an English scientist cleverly devised a contraption to catch whatever was wafting about in the air. An insect net was constructed to open and close at various altitudes and was attached to a box kite. Flown over the playing fields of his university, the net trapped 839 insects in over a hundred hours of flying time at heights varying from 150 to 2,000 feet. The scientist was astonished to find that they were all small, light-bodied insects whose powers of flight were weak or nonexistent: small flies, lice, and the like. Other studies using airplanes to trap insects at various altitudes have led to an estimate that within a column of air one mile square, starting fifty feet from the ground and rising to fourteen thousand feet, there will be about twenty-five million insects. Add to these the pollen, seeds, spores, bacteria, and man-made pollutants, and one may wonder that we do not see air as a solid.

The unusual densities of the three insect groups that we have discussed make their relationship to allergy definable, but hundreds, perhaps thousands of other insect species, for the most part unnoticed by ourselves, live and die in our environment and affect the hypersensitive. We often cannot draw breath without inhaling bits of insects, their dried secretions, or feces. This is unsettling enough, but the thought that we also consume all this in our food is downright revolting. Yet it is so, and we have not yet devised a way to make our edibles free of these products of nature's prodigal way. Insects also like to dine on what we consider human fare, and this ensures that they will be with us always in one form or another. The federal government recognizes this and so allows for a certain amount of insect debris in food products. Beyond and above this set limit, the food is considered contaminated. The World Health Organization has estimated that millions of tons of the world's grains and rice have been insect-contaminated annually. It seems ironic that on the one hand we are considering insects as a possible source of edible protein while on the other we are upset when they become so widely incorporated into our foodstuffs. Obviously we prefer to choose the insects we dine upon. I expect there are few individuals who would care for fried cockroach.

If one is looking for a common source of food contamination other than the fecund fly, the cockroach is it. It pains one's human sensibilities to think that, if we do away with the human species through the medium of massively murderous wars, the roach and the rat will be our most likely successors. The prospect that this gruesome pair could be the next rulers of the world ought to keep us peaceful if nothing else will.

The cockroach has been eminently successful down the corridors of time. There are about 3,500 species running about. While they most resemble beetles, they are actually cousins to crickets, grasshoppers, and locusts. The only places on earth that roaches have not inhabited so far are the ice-bound regions of the Arctic and Antarctic. From their very ubiquitousness and their great numbers one might believe that cockroaches are already sovereign. Many a homemaker would agree, for the cocky cockroach is difficult to eradicate once established.

Although we are apt to think of cockroaches as invaders of our homes, the truth is that most species prefer to make it in the wild. They make their living as scavengers upon fungi and plant and animal debris, which is a reasonably dignified way of life for an insect. Of the fifty or so species that abound in our land only five invade our homes. Somewhere along the line they seem to have developed a sweet tooth for sugar and starch, although they apparently will eat just about anything—paper, books, clothing, shoes, even bones. Not only do they race about with dirty feet over uncovered foodstuffs during the dark of the night but, worse yet, they also have habit of vomiting half-digested meals, mixed with a smelly secretion, and depositing feces wherever they go.

Cockroaches come in various sizes and in varying shades of brown and black. Their flat, shiny bodies, fronted by long, slender antennaei, are easy to identify. Most cockroach species are able to fly but prefer to scuttle, perhaps because they are so good at it. Any housewife who has turned on the kitchen light suddenly at night will attest to their speed. While they breed and flourish best in unsanitary conditions, it is possible for them to enter a restaurant or the most immaculate of homes in food cartons, grocery bags, and the like. Once they can get a cockroach toehold, they multiply overnight, or so it often seems.

Living as they do and possessing such gruesome habits, it seemed impossible that cockroaches did not transmit disease. Yet it took researchers a long time to find out what exactly they did transmit. Finally they were clearly indicted during an unpleasant outbreak of a Salmonella strain in a pediatric hospital in Brussels. Children continued to get sick, even after they were isolated from all other patients and every possible step had been taken to avoid transmission of the bacteria. The one exception to the measures that were taken was the presence of the cockroaches, which continued to invade the wards at night to crawl over the clothing, the bedding, and the children themselves. Laboratory studies of the roaches demonstrated that the Salmonella bacteria were present, so measures were taken to destroy them (and high time too, I may add). As soon as the cockroaches were eradicated, the cases of Salmonella declined and then ceased.

It is now known that cockroaches can also carry cholera, anthrax, tuberculosis, and a number of other disease organisms. They deposit these in our food and water with their vomit and their feces and track them onto whatever they race across, be it food, bedding, or human skin. Incidentally, they have even been known to nibble the fingers, toenails, and surrounding skin of the sick, the sleeping, and infants.

It is the vomit, the feces, and the particles of cockroach bodies left behind in food that most affect the allergic. Some individuals are highly sensitive to such things. That is allergically speaking—I am sure most people would exhibit a more general kind of sensitivity if they knew such things existed in our daily fare.

There are other insects, although perhaps none is quite so repulsive, that get into our foodstuffs. Weevils, moths, beetles, mites—in toto or just their debris—are often ingested, more often perhaps than most of us realize. The reader who has reached this point in the book may consider himself under seige: the world out there may appear alive with bugs, beetles, and bees ready to sting, bite, or just plain contaminate. But before you rush out to buy a bomb or a spray or some powder to poison the pests, pause long enough to read the last chapter: caution is the watchword.

READER'S GUIDE TO INHALANT AND INGESTANT ALLERGY:

Know the enemy:

In diagnosing cases of inhalant or ingestant allergy, it is necessary only to know that one or more insect species abound in the air or in food, since a number of species are capable of causing allergy symptoms when inhaled and, less commonly, ingested. Thus if an individual suffers from respiratory problems only in a mayfly region and during the time when mayflies swarm, it is probable that the mayfly is the cause. Suspicion is a number-one factor in diagnosis.

What to do if allergic to inhaled insects:

If skin tests demonstrate that the individual is allergic to an insect species that exists in large numbers in the area, hyposensitization may be helpful, depending upon the insect species involved, but it is generally not as successful as with, say, allergy to pollen.

Medications consist of antihistamines and, if wheezing develops, oral bronchodilators. In severer asthmatic reactions adrenaline may be employed.

How individuals allergic to insect debris in the air can avoid problems:

They can wear masks or respirators when working outdoors or when they are outdoors for any length of time, especially if their symptoms coincide with seasonal insect swarms such as those of the mayfly and the caddis fly. Often, however, relief rests simply with getting out of the area until the swarming is well over.

225

INGESTANT AND INHALANT ALLERGIES

INGESTANT AND INHALANT ALLERGIES

What to do if allergic to insects ingested:

There is not much one can do about foodstuffs contaminated during the course of their production except avoid the products when they are recognized as, or suspected to be, the cause of allergy symptoms.

One can rid the home of such contaminating insects as cockroaches. Several insecticides on the market are effective against most of the home-loving roaches. They must be applied in the proper places, for instance, under sinks and in cracks, especially in the kitchen and bathroom areas; behind window and door frames and baseboards; in the backs of closets and bookshelves; above cupboards; under chairs and tables; around the edges of drawers; and even behind pictures on the wall.

Whatever insecticides are used, care must be taken that toxic materials do not get onto eating utensils or food. Plain boric-acid powder spread carefully on cockroach runs and in hiding places is an effective eradicator. Periodically applied in the proper areas, it is safe to use and can clear the home of roaches. A dusting device is the most effective means to apply it.

22
How to Kill Insect Pests Without Killing Yourself

As the 1970's drew to a close Nova Scotia authorities canceled an ambitious spruce-budworm spraying project in their forests when a mysterious outbreak of an uncommon but highly fatal disease was discovered among children in an area of neighboring New Brunswick extensively sprayed in the past. The illness, Reyes syndrome, is viral, but a three-year study of this particular outbreak suggested that chemicals used in the antibudworm pesticide had interacted with ordinary, run-of-the-mill viruses to produce the highly lethal syndrome. It was not a consequence of the use of pesticides that anyone foresaw, and it is probable that only the death of children would ever have suggested such an interaction of chemicals and viruses. The incident illuminates clearly the kind of Russian roulette that we have been playing with pesticides during the last half century or so. There is an ever-present chance that a pesticide we employ against the insect world will backfire to do us far more harm than good.

We realized this odd dilemma when Rachel Carson's book *Silent Spring* dropped like a block-busting bomb on our technological complacency. The book not only shattered a good many nerves but also exposed a great uncertainty and a good bit of human stupidity. For the first time we saw what we were doing with substances that were toxic not only to plant and animal life but to our own as well. We were aghast, as well we might be. It can be argued that the pendulum has swung too far, that we have become too antipesticide, but speaking as a medical man, I believe that it is better that we err on the side of too much caution rather than not enough. As Rachel Carson showed us, many toxic substances not only persist in the environment for many years but also magnify through the food chain. As a physician I have a paramount interest in human health, and I think it probable that we played a dangerous game in the past, and am not totally reassured that we are not still gambling.

Yet there have to be trade-offs in life. We have a growing problem in trying to raise enough food to feed a hungry and overpopulated world, and starvation is as much a hazard to human health as cancer. I can hope that we will have the restraint and the intelligence to employ pesticides only when we absolutely must. Apples not quite unblemished, vegetables not quite perfect are to be preferred over a lingering, painful death from cancer and permanent brain damage among the vulnerable young, or chronic invalidism. One thing is certain: we can make our choices only when we really know what sort of trade-off we are making; we must be able to weigh benefits against hazards fairly, or our choices are likely to be irrational and risky.

Let us begin by understanding our definitions. For instance, the term pesticides includes toxic agents such as insecticides, herbicides, fungicides, rodenticides, nematocides, and arachnicides. There are almost 100,000 of these agents registered with the United States government, based on approximately 1,000 different chemicals in various formulations. The registered agents include some cosmetics, drugs, and cleaning agents—in fact, any agent that is considered necessary to our lives but poses a possible health hazard. The only two classifications of pesticides that concern us in this book are insecticides and arachnicides, or spider poisons.

The usual methods of applying insecticides and arachnicides are spraying, dusting, or baiting. The first two methods involve the greatest potential exposure to toxic substances for us as well as the target insects, not to mention other animal life, including beneficial species. It has been estimated, for instance, that as much as 70 percent of the spray put down by airplanes either misses the intended target or drifts away from it. Dusting by ground machinery may be equally unconfined. Sprays and dusts not only are carried about by air currents but also frequently find their way into water courses, be they lakes, streams, or rivers. Thus they find their way some distance from the original site of application.

One of the great paradoxes in our use of insecticides and pesticides is that the more we use, the more we have to use to achieve the same effect. The target insects develop resistance to our sprays, and the chemicals become proportionately less effective as a result. Also nature is far more complex than we give her credit for being: she has so interwoven the various life forms that we cannot rid ourselves of what we consider pests without also doing away with beneficial life forms, some of which help us survive even though we may be unaware of their aid. Predators of pest insects generally exist in far smaller numbers than their prey. When we spray or dust to kill the pests, we also kill the predators, but the latter do not bounce back with the strength and rapidity of the pests. Thus the result of our application of an insecticide can be the direct opposite of what we wished to achieve. We kill off the pests, yes, but enough survive to carry on, and since we killed off their predators, the survivors' population mushrooms undisturbed, forcing us to spray once again. As the cycle repeats, we apply more and more toxic chemicals.

Figures tell the story. We humans used 40 percent more pesticides of various kinds in 1971 than we did five years earlier, and the figures appear to be rising still. Farmers spread about 494 million pounds of pesticides—almost $1 billion worth—in 1971 to battle bugs, weeds, and rats. There is no denying that that is a lot of toxic stuff bandied about in the environment, especially when we note that farmers accounted for only 59 percent of the pesticides used in that year.

The story of DDT is by now an old tale. A chlorinated hydrocarbon, DDT was hailed as a miracle insecticide during

World War II. It did yeoman duty saving the lives of refugees, survivors of concentration camps, soldiers, and the ill-nourished populations of Europe following the war. The great scourges of war—the infectious diseases such as bubonic plague and typhus—were kept at bay. But within a few years it was discovered that insects were becoming resistant to DDT. Worse still, DDT seemed to have spread across the world—in the air, the water, food, animals, and us. We found that we store it in body fat, and finally, many years after its introduction into the environment, we have found that it has definite health effects. Studies of workers in DDT plants (where, of course, exposure was unusally great) showed that early symptoms of DDT poisoning were headache, dizziness, muscular impairment, loss of appetite, and general feelings of not being well. One study demonstrated that a group of DDT workers had a high rate of liver, heart, and neurological problems. Laboratory experiments with animals concluded that long-term exposure could induce cancer. By the end of 1972 the general use of DDT had been banned in the United States.

The DDT pattern has been repeated with other pesticides. We find a miracle insecticide. We use it liberally. Insects grow resistant, and predators are decimated. We use more and more of the poison. Suddenly, to our horror we find that the stuff can affect us too. We ban it and start over again with a new insecticide. Fortunately, there are people who are experimenting with other ways—better ways. We are moving toward biological controls, and perhaps just in time, for the scales on which we must weigh the cost-benefit aspects of insecticides are wobbly affairs, and none of us can be sure that the weights themselves are true.

The sometimes accidental way in which we learn about the hazards of insecticide chemicals can also be unnerving. Kepone is a prime example. An episode in Hopewell, Virginia, in 1975 made us suddenly aware that kepone could be exceedingly toxic when a number of workers in a chemical plant were hospitalized. We learned that it can turn healthy individuals into invalids, possibly for life. Now kepone is turning up in strange places, sometimes far removed from the

Hopewell area where the James River was contaminated. Recently the Environmental Protection Agency discovered that the milk of some southeastern mothers contained traces of it. It has been suggested that, since the widely used Mirex, which was employed to control fire ants in the Southeast, degenerates to form kepone (among other substances) kepone may have migrated into the food chain. Research is under way to track down the source of the kepone traces.

The problem of the widely used insecticide Mirex and the fire ant is a perfect example of the dilemma in which we so often find ourselves when employing insecticides: in spite of increasing applications of Mirex throughout the South, fire ants have increased and spread to new areas; yet Mirex is the only toxic substance that has been at all effective. Nevertheless, since it poses a definite health risk, its use has been phased out.

The fire-ant sting is extremely painful and can be serious, even fatal. But we do not know what those traces of kepone in mothers' milk may do to the babies or even eventually to the mothers themselves.

Methods for massive insect control began in the 1800s with reasoned advice to farmers whose production of large areas of single crops had caused the various destructive insect species to multiply. The original agricultural wisdom was to lure the insects and crush them by hand. Then a bright new idea arrived: spray the crops with whale oil, and when the insect pests slip off to the ground, stamp them. In the middle of the century someone developed a horse-drawn roller device that could move through potato fields knocking potato bugs loose and then squashing them under the roller. But the battle had only just begun. Paris green arrived on the scene, followed closely by London Purple. Both contained arsenic. They enjoyed a temporary, if colorful, popularity, for by the end of the century farmers favored lead arsenate. This last insecticide reigned until DDT arrived during World War II.

In fact, arsenic became so popular during the nineteenth century that it was widely employed in such things as cosmetics, paints, wallpaper, wrappings for food, candles, materials, and even in the coloring dyes for candy. Arsenic was scattered about the environment and into the works of mankind with utter abandon. Yet perhaps we really should not shake our heads in wonder at such incredible blindness to the dangers of a toxic substance, for we have just recently realized that DDT, kepone, PCB, and perhaps many other toxic substances have been loosed in much the same manner and in the same ignorance of consequences. Sad to relate, in the nineteenth century as now, the medical community was unaware of the possibilities for disaster from arsenic poisoning. Chronic cases kept surfacing, and there were fatalities. Land became so saturated that cattle pastured on it years later keeled over dead. Yet arsenic compounds disappeared from the scene only because they were replaced by the synthetic organic insecticides. DDT came along and rescued the world from arsenic—and also replaced it as the brand-new threat to bug and man both and to all sorts of other animals.

The two main groups of organic pesticides are the chlorinated hydrocarbons and the organophosphates. The best-known chlorinated hydrocarbon is DDT. Among other members of this group are lindane, chlordane, endrin, aldrin, benzene hexachloride, and isodrin. Although the government has banned some of these compounds, the damage has been done—as the story of the bats of Carlsbad Caverns clearly illustrates. Bats are great natural insect-control resources. They consume insects literally by the ton. It has been estimated that a good-sized bat colony of about 250,000 inhabitants dines upon two to four tons of insects every night. Unhappily, chlorinated hydrocarbons have put the bat population into a steep decline. Many species of insects have become resistant to DDT, but the unfortunate bats have stored in their body fat the DDT that they have consumed while dining on insects laced with the stuff. The hypothesis is that, when the bats undertake long flights and the stored fat is metabolized, enough DDT is released to kill them. We humans should take note, for most of us also have stored DDT (and other organic toxic substances) in our body fat. It is conceivable that we have phased DDT out of the picture just in time: a few more years of extensive use and the Olympics might have become a charnel house, not to mention Saturday-afternoon football games.

In the organophosphate group are such insecticides as parathion and Malathion. They are close cousins to nerve gas—a battle tool developed during World War II for possible use in removing a good bit of the human species from the face of the earth. While Malathion is deadly to insects, fortunately for us mammals, we possess an enzyme that destroys the chemical in our systems. Parathion, however, can kill us right along with the insects it has been designed for, and it has. People have died when this very toxic substance has been spilled or has leaked into food products. In less dramatic but nonetheless unfortunate cases, agricultural workers have suffered chronic illness from working in fields treated with this insecticide.

A third group of chemical insecticides, the carbamates (of which Sevin is one), are generally less toxic and less persistent in the environment. Some of the compounds have been highly effective against aphids and houseflies.

Inorganic and synthetic organic insecticides are not the only ones that pose problems. The botanical insecticides, while less toxic, can still be hazardous to human health. The best known of the botanicals are pyrethrum and rotenone. Pyrethrum is manufactured from powdered flowers—colorful members of the genus Chrysanthemum. While the botanicals are safer to use than most of the other insecticides, they are still poisons and must be handled with care.

In fact, handling with care is one prong of the two-pronged approach that we must take to the use of toxic substances in the control of insect pests if we are not to make the cure worse than the problem. The other prong would seem self-evident, but if past history is anything to judge by, is far from being so: it is the simple rule that toxic substance should be applied only when absolutely necessary and when no other way can be found to control the insects in question.

We have recently become aware that, when we employ toxic substances to attack any form of life, all life is potentially threatened in one way or another, and fortunately we have been casting about for other methods of controlling insects. Ideas range from keeping pet toads in the garden to sterilizing tens of thousands of male insects and turning them loose to check the insect population explosion. Both of these ideas work. A pet toad is likely to consume several hundred insects a night, which adds up to thousands during the summer months. He or she, as the case may be, should be encouraged to stick around, although toads, like everything else in this life, have a drawback: they tend to relish those precious earthworms as well as the insect pests.

One of the best examples of what sterilization and the release of the sterile males can accomplish is the all-but-total eradication of the screw worm from the southeastern part of the United States and the great reduction in its depredations in the West. In the case of the screwworm millions, even billions, of male flies are raised and then sterilized, often by suspension in canisters in a lead-lined chamber where they are exposed to radiation by cobalt 60. When they are relased in screwworm areas, they mate but produce infertile eggs that never develop. If enough are released in proportion to the number of normal males in the region, the screwworm population begins to drop and may disappear altogether. There are also chemicals to sterilize insects that are reared in the laboratory for release or reached with chemical bait in the wild. Research is still being done to ascertain the most effective compounds and, we can hope, the safest.

Somewhat along these lines are the new growth regulators, which are discussed briefly in Chapter 8 above. The hormones that regulate the transformation of various insects from the larva through the pupa to the adult state have been constructed that mimic the hormones so well that they can keep the insects in an intermediate state and prevent their reaching maturity. Among other things this means that the insect cannot reproduce. The application of growth regulators as an insecticide can be a bit tricky, however, since some insects are most destructive in the larva stage. To arrest their development at this point would increase their depredations considerably. The most effective use of growth regulators, therefore, will probably be against such insects as the bean beetle and the mosquito, which do most of their damage as adults.

In the same vein as the juvenile-hormone regulator is another growth regulator that affects the development of chitin, the horny substance contained in insect shells. The shells of insects treated with this chemical during the larva stage may be so weakened that they break or are deformed, and the insect is hindered from moving about and feeding. These options sound like something straight from sci-fi, creating as they do insect Frankensteins and other monsters.

Less like, science-fiction, synthetic sex attractants, or pheromones, have been developed for specific insect species. Females of various species, and sometimes the males, give off a powerful sex pheromone that can be detected by insects of the opposite sex several miles away. This technique so far has been used mainly to bait traps to estimate infestations in a given area. It is thought that, if widely used, it will be an effective control measure. Its disadvantages are that it entraps only one sex of a species and is specific to only one species.

Bacterial insecticides have also received attention lately. The first success in this field was milky spore, a bacteria that goes after Japanese beetles as handily as a flock of pheasants. It kills the beetles in the larva stage. Other bacterial products are being researched and may soon be in use. Drawbacks are several. For instance, they are comparatively slow acting, and they may lose their efficacy during weather extremes. Their advantages are considerable. They are insect-specific and do not harm other animals, including ourselves. They do no damage to plants. As far as is known, insects develop no resistance to them.

Of course, nature has her own way of controlling insects. One of the cleverest is the predator. Insect predators destroy vast quantities of their fellow insects, and any gardener with his garden's best interests at heart will not only pamper toads

INSECTICIDES

but also stock his plot with praying mantises and ladybugs. They are voracious consumers of aphids, grasshoppers, and other destructive pests.

Man has also designed some clever insect traps to lure insects to their doom. Some simply trap the pests. Others trap and poison them. Some zap them electronically. Often all that is needed is a sticky, alluring bait or a light to draw the insects to their destruction. The old flypapers that used to hang messily from the ceilings of grocery stores were no things of beauty, but they caught flies. Bait pails of a mixture of sugar water and fermenting molasses, hung about in trees or bushes or even sunk in the ground, often caught their share of insects, which tried to take a sip but ended up with a slip into the gooey drink.

We have some old-fashioned insecticides that may smell rotten but are not at all toxic—frequently not even toxic to their targets, who seem to hasten away from the odor more than the poison. For instance, centuries ago the Egyptians found that garlic could chase bugs from their crops. Organic gardeners have resurrected several recipes for garlic sprays that are guaranteed to make the garden unfit for insects and perhaps for the gardener himself. They include such things as chopped-up onions, red pepper, cloves of garlic, chives, leeks, soap powder, and water. Recipes for some of these natural insecticides are reproduced in **Appendix I.**

READER'S GUIDE TO INSECTICIDES:

How to use toxic insecticides:

- Read the label on the container. Know exactly what is in the insecticide and exactly how it should be used, whether it is a spray, a dust, a liquid, or bait pellets.
- Follow the directions to the letter.
- Keep the container until all danger of accidental poisoning is past. In the case of an accident information on the

236

label may be vital to the doctor because the antidote for one compound may be the wrong treatment for another.

- Avoid inhalation of or skin contact with the insecticide. Avoid exposure of any great duration. Wear gloves, and if you are applying the insecticide to a large area, it is safer to use a respirator and protective clothing.
- Never apply an insecticide where food or drinking water is exposed, whether for human beings or animals.
- Wash after each application with soap and water. If the insecticide comes in contact with the skin, wash the area thoroughly with soap and water.
- If you must wash out the spray or other equipment, do so where no animal or human being can come in accidental contact with the chemicals.
- Always store insecticides in safe, locked places with the labels intact. Never store them in unmarked containers, in which the contents may be mistaken.
- Bury empty insecticide containers under at least two feet of earth or, if this is in agreement with local practices, wrap household-type insecticide containers in plastic bags or several thicknesses of newspaper and dispose of them in the trash. The container should be closed as tightly as possible, even taped shut, to prevent leakage.
- Know what to do in case of accidental poisoning. Immediate emergency treatment measures are printed on the label.

Find out which insecticides can be used safely:

It would be unwise to recommend specific insecticides, since often what is considered safe today is banned tomorrow. Under the law insecticide containers are labeled, depending on the potential toxicity of the contents, in the following manner:

- *Highly toxic* insecticide labels must show "DANGER," "POISON," a skull and crossbones, and antidote statement, "Call physician immediately," and "Keep out of reach of children."

- *Moderately toxic* insecticide labels must show "WARN-ING," "Keep out of reach of children," but no antidote statement is required.
- Insecticides of a *low order of toxicity* must be labeled "CAUTION" and "Keep out of reach of children," but no antidote statement is required.
- Insecticides that are *comparatively free from danger* bear no warning, caution, or antidote statement, but cannot make unqualified safety claims and are labeled, "Keep out of reach of children."

How you can find out what insecticides are safest:

- Many localities have poison-control centers with current information about not only the chemicals themselves but also the correct treatment of accidental poisonings and other problems.
- State health departments may have up-to-date information.
- The county agricultural extension agent is a good source of information and of help in the techniques and times of proper insecticide application.
- The Environmental Protection Agency, through its Washington office or its regional offices, is another source of information.

How accidental poisonings occur:

- Insecticide mists, fumes, or dusts can be inhaled. Smoking during application can increase the danger. Also, if cigarettes or tobacco become contaminated with the insecticide, poisoning can occur through inhalation.
- Insecticides can be ingested. Dusts and sprays can be ingested during application. Food and drinking water can become contaminated. The insecticide can be trans-

ferred from contaminated clothing or the hands. Containers can be used for insecticide storage and then mistakenly for food or drink. Insecticide can be accidentally drunk from unlabeled bottles or jars.

• Insecticide poisoning can occur through contact with the skin because of accidental spills on skin or clothing, use of the spray in wind, insecticide dusts settling on the skin, splash or spray of the chemicals during mixing, contact with treated plants or other surfaces too soon after application of the insecticide, and children playing with discarded insecticide containers.

INSECTICIDES

Appendix A
Emergency! Symptoms of Systemic Reaction to Insect Stings or Bites

Early systemic reaction symptoms:

Itching around the eyes
Dry, hacking cough
Widespread hives
Constriction of chest and throat
Wheezing
Nausea
Abdominal pain
Vomiting
Dizziness

More severe systemic symptoms:

Difficulty in breathing
Hoarseness and thickened speech
Difficulty in swallowing
Confusion
A sense of impending disaster

Anaphylactic shock symptoms:

Cyanosis (bluish, purplish, or grayish coloring of the skin)
Reduced blood pressure
Incontinence
Unconsciousness
Death

Treatment:

- Act quickly if any of these symptoms is present.
- Scrape out the insect stinger, if one is present, with a fingernail or a knife.

- Apply ice to the sting or bite site if possible.
- If you or the victim possess an insect-sting kit, administer the epinephrine (or adrenaline) and other measures in the kit as directed. Then take the victim as quickly as possible to the nearest medical help. Do not rely on the epinephrine to do more than stave off the systemic reaction long enough to get the victim to a physician or to a hospital emergency room.
- If you use the tourniquet contained in the insect kit, be sure to loosen it every three to five minutes and remove it when symptoms appear to be under control.

Appendix B
The Insect-Sting Kit

Several types of insect sting kits are on the market, but in most, if not all, states they can be obtained only with a doctor's prescription. I advise my patients to obtain the kit:

- If they have had any of the symptoms of a generalized systemic reaction listed in appendix A.
- If they have previously had a local reaction to an insect sting that was marked by considerable swelling that covered two or more joints or was clearly abnormal for other reasons.

One type of kit contains a preloaded, two-dose sterile syringe of measured epinephrine, a tourniquet, antihistamine tablets, and an alcohol swab in a sealed packet. Its advantages are that it is easy to administer the epinephrine since it is already premeasured and within the syringe. Its disadvantage is that, if a second dose of epinephrine is needed, the syringe may have become contaminated. Some physicians state that the epinephrine in this type of sting kit often deteriorates within a year or so, although according to the manufacturer, this situation has improved. Another kit contains two sterile unloaded syringes and two sealed ampules of epinephrine, a tourniquet, an alcohol swab, warning medical-tag information, and information on how to avoid stinging insects. It does not contain antihistamines or other medications. The advantage to this kit is that, with two sterile needles, if a second dose is needed before the victim can be gotten to medical help, there is far less risk of contamination during the second injection. Also, since antihistamines or other medications are not included in the kit, the victim is less likely to settle for these measures, which are actually ineffective, in lieu of giving himself an injection. Epinephrine is the only drug that will stabilze a person during a fulminating systemic reaction. The manufacturers of this kit also claim that the epinephrine will remain stable far longer in sealed ampules than in syringes. The main disadvantage of this type of kit—and it is a big disadvantage—is that a nervous, frightened victim who must inject himself quickly with the epinephrine is going to have great difficulty breaking open the sealed ampules and filling the syringes. Even under the best of circumstances such a maneuver, which may be easy and simple for the experienced, is not so for the inexperienced. Nor could I advise that this kit be used for children, since the syringes are ungraded, and a child's dose of epinephrine must be less than that of an adult. The syringe must be marked to obtain that lesser dose. Whichever type of kit one chooses, I recommend that an individual who is allergic to insects or, for that matter, severely allergic to anything— food, inhalants, or drugs—obtain three kits in order to keep one in the home, one in the glove compartment of his car, and one on his person whenever and wherever he may encounter stinging insects, or whatever his nemesis may be.

Appendix C
Medical Warning Tags
and Bracelets

Several brands of medical neck tags and bracelets are on the market. I recommend that anyone severely allergic to insect bites or stings always wear one, for time is of the essence when a severe allergic reaction occurs. A misdiagnosis could spell the difference between life and death. Since loss of consciousness frequently occurs during such a reaction, an attending physician needs all the help he can get. This is especially true when the reaction is of an emergency nature and there is no time to contact the patient's regular physician. The special feature of the Medic Alert Foundation tags or bracelets is that the foundation maintains files on everyone who purchases its products and operates a headquarters office twenty-four hours a day. This enables the physician who is confronted with an unconscious victim to call collect to obtain the patient's medical history. The tag also alerts the physician if the patient is allergic to insects, drugs, foods, or whatever, making his task of diagnosis not only easier but swifter. The address of the Medic Alert Foundation is Turlock, California 95380. Most pharmacies carry the foundation's tags and bracelets along with complete information and medical-history cards to be filled out and sent in.

Appendix D
When to See Your Physician

A physician should be consulted whenever an insect sting results in marked swelling, especially if the dwelling covers more than two joints (for example, a sting on a finger that results in swelling beyond the wrist). Consult a physician if any of the following symptoms of a systemic reaction occur:

Itching around the eyes
Dry, hacking cough
Wheezing and breathing difficulties
Widespread hives
Nausea, vomiting, and abdominal pain
Dizziness
Constriction in throat and chest
Thickened speech
Difficulty in swallowing

Anyone stung in the throat or eye area should see a physician as quickly as possible. A sting in the mouth and throat area can cause sufficient swelling to make breathing difficult. A sting close to the eye may cause damage to the eye itself either from the effects of a local reaction or because the stinger works its way into the eye through the lid. In the case of insect stings or bites, be alert for signs of secondary infection. Such signs are:

Redness
Inflammation
Swelling
Discharge of fluid
Some degree of pain

A doctor should always be consulted at the first signs of such symptoms.

Appendix E
Measures to Avoid
Bites and Stings

To minimize contact with stinging insects:

- Begin seek-and-destroy missions against Hymenoptera hives, nests, and colonies early in the spring and continue to search the home and its environs periodically during the warm months of the year to destroy nests before they get difficult to handle. Let someone who is not allergic handle the chore of destruction.
- Avoid attracting Hymenoptera by smelling or looking like a flower. Avoid the use of perfumes, sweet-smelling shampoos and soaps, and the like from April until the first heavy freeze in the fall. Do not wear flowery prints, bright colors, jewelry, or the like outdoors.
- Do not run barefoot during the warm weather months. In areas where Hymenoptera are likely to be encountered, wear long pants and long sleeves and keep long hair tied up or covered.
- Stay away from clover patches, gardens full of blossoms, blossoming trees, and other areas where Hymenoptera are busy making a living. Let someone else pick the flowers, trim the hedges, mow the lawns.
- Be wary around garbage cans, littered picnic areas, and trees where fruit has fallen and is rotting, for these are favorite places for scavenger Hymenoptera, such as the yellow jackets.
- Keep an insecticide spray can (non-pressurized) in the glove compartment of the car (right beside your insect-sting kit) to use against invading Hymenoptera.
- If you find yourself in imminent danger of being stung, retreat slowly. Do not panic. Do not, above all, swat at your attackers, since this may anger them enough to sting. If retreat seems impossible, lie flat on the ground and cover your head and face with your arms.

Appendix E

To minimize contact with biting insects:

- Avoid their hideouts. For instance, black widows like dark corners, chiggers abound in brush, and ticks like to lurk along pathways. The preferences of other species are discussed in the preceding chapters.
- Wear protective clothing, especially gloves, when you must invade what could be the domain of the biters.
- Use repellents as outlined in **Appendix F.**
- Wear light-colored clothing and try not to sweat.
- Eliminate the breeding places of the biters insofar as is possible.
- Use insecticides if and when you must. **See Appendix G.**

To minimize contact with both stingers and biters:

- Keep yard and home clean and free of debris, piles of rubbish, lumber stacks, and the like. Keep the lawn mowed and the brush cut down and pick up fruit from beneath trees.
- Do not leave food or garbage out to attract insects.
- Do not eat Popsicles, ice-cream cones, watermelon, and other fare outdoors that is attractive to insects.
- Always shake out clothing and bedding that has not been used for some time; it can harbor wasps, spiders, and the like.
- Keep pets free of fleas, ticks, and mites. When powdering, spraying, or bathing pets, include their bedding and their favorite curling-up places, in the treatment.

Appendix F
Repellents and How to Use Them

Chemical repellents:

Chemical repellents are intended not to kill insects but simply to send them packing. Such repellents come in sprays, powders, lotions, or solid sticks to be rubbed on. One general type is conveniently labeled "personal repellent" and is designed to be applied to the body or clothing of the individual himself. Foggers and sprayers that combine an insecticide to kill with a repelling chemical are not for use on the person but are considered area repellents. The most effective ingredient of chemical repellents is diethyltoluamide. It may be called Deet, Metadelphene, Delphene, Detamide, or Det.

Johnson Wax, the manufacturer of repellents, offers the following advice (which I quote with the company's permission):

Where to use
[Repellents] are most effective when applied to all exposed skin as well as to clothing. . . .

Where not to use
Do not apply to articles made from spandex, rayon, Dynel, or Verel as . . . [repellents] can damage these fibers. Also, do not use personal insect repellents on tents and other camping equipment or on fishing gear. Insect repellents should not be sprayed into air or on surfaces. Avoid spilling or spraying . . . on furniture finishes, plastics or painted surfaces. Care should be taken not to get . . . [the] product into the eyes, on the lips, on scratches or other areas of broken skin. Do not expose treated surfaces to fire or flame.

How to use
A. *Aerosol:*
  1. Holding container as upright as possible and about 6 to 8 inches away, spray clothing and/or skin with a slow, sweeping motion until slightly moist. Spread the material with your hands to insure complete coverage of all exposed skin.
  2. Apply to face and neck by spraying into the hand and rubbing product onto skin. Avoid application to eyes and lips.

249

B. *Lotion:*
  1. Pour product into palm of hand.
  2. Rub hands together, then spread product lightly on skin or over clothing.

NOTE: Complete coverage of all exposed skin is important as insects may seek out even the smallest unprotected area. Reapply repellent as needed, especially if insects are persistent and after swimming or perspiring heavily.

Special tips

Directions for various types of repellents and insecticides vary with the product. Each is formulated for a specific use and should be used and handled in the way intended by the manufacturer. Always read the directions on the package before each use and note any safety precautions for proper handling. Use good judgment when storing these products and keep them where they will be out of the reach of children.

A personal repellent should be applied only to skin and clothing as directed on the label. Spraying personal repellent into the air would do nothing to discourage biting pests since repellents do not kill insects. An insecticide should be used to destroy flying or crawling insects. Two basic types are available and each has a different purpose. Space sprays are formulated with a special knock-down ingredient. When sprayed into the air, they kill flying insects on contact. To control crawling insects like ants or roaches, a residual insecticide should be used. Residual products are applied to surfaces where bugs crawl. Their long-lasting effect destroys insects once they have come in contact with the treated surface.

As I noted in Chapter 12 in the discussion of chiggers, the liberal use of flowers of sulfur (powdered sulfur) in shoes and on socks and pants legs discourages these pests. The heat of the body transforms the inactive sulfur to a sulphide, which chiggers apparently do not care for.

Oral drugs that repel insects:

Some people, including some physicians, swear by thiamine, or vitamin B^1, taken orally, as an effective repellent, especially against mosquitoes. It has been suggested that it affects the nature of the individual's sweat to make it repulsive to mosquitoes coming in for a bite. Although there are many testimonials to this vitamin's effectiveness as a repellent against mosquitoes, no real research has been done, as far as I know, to determine the validity of personal experience or to demonstrate how the vitamin works as a repellent.

Other protective measures:

One Maine doctor in the heart of the blackfly country instructs mothers of young children to smear their skin with baby oil before turning them out to play during blackfly season in order to keep the fly from contact with the tender young skin. Meat tenderizer containing papaya applied to a sting is said to relieve pain.

Appendix G
Insecticides

Four main groups of insecticides are in wide use today: the chlorinated hydrocarbons (which include DDT), the organophosphates (which include parathion), the carbamates, and the botanicals, such as pyrethrum. With their kind permission, let me quote the Johnson Wax company's brochure on the home use of insecticides:

Airborne insecticides

Airborne insecticides are released into the air to rid an area of flying insects. Many products of this type are packaged in aerosol cans or other spray containers and are often referred to as space sprays. Another type comes in the form of a solid material treated with insecticide that provides continuous control of flying insects. Both types are convenient to use, as they are self-contained packages that require no mixing or handling of the product. They are released in the proper amount for efficient control of insect pests.

Aerosol airborne insecticides often contain pyrethrin, a fast-working ingredient that causes very rapid knockdown and paralysis of flying insects. Pyrethrin is a natural insecticide extracted from the pyrethrum flower, a daisy-like plant of the chrysanthemum family. It is an effective, fast-acting killer for most common insect pests. It works effectively for a short time and then dissipates when exposed to sunlight and air. Pyrethrin can be synergized to boost its own effectiveness and that of other product ingredients, resulting in more efficient products for insect control. Also, science has brought us man-made pyrethroids which are just as effective as pyrethrin, and are more readily available.

Special tips

When using aerosol airborne insecticides to clear a room of flying insects, best results will be obtained if all windows and doors in the room are closed prior to treatment. Leave the room closed for 15 minutes after using the insecticide to be sure all insects are destroyed.

Most airborne insecticides can be safely used in food preparation areas, but cover any exposed food, dishes and cooking utensils while spraying. Fish bowls should also be covered and birds removed from the room. If eating or cooking utensils have been left uncovered while using an insecticide, wash them in hot water with detergent before using them again. Discard any food exposed during spray treatment.

Aerosol insecticides are very cold as they come from the container due to rapid evaporation of the propellent which creates a chilling effect. When using such a product to kill chewing and sucking insects on plants, hold the container at least 3 feet from the foliage. From this distance, the product mist will drift over the leaves, carrying the insecticide with it, but the cold temperature from the evaporating propellent will not reach the plant. If the product is applied at a closer range, it could cause frostbite. Leaves may turn brown and fall off, although the damage is usually not permanent and new growth should appear before too long.

Fleas are sometimes noticed after the home has been vacant for a time, usually after a vacation. Fleas live and breed in dust and lint, but need a blood meal to exist. A cat or dog is usually the host and if the pet is removed from the home for a time, any fleas present become more active as they search for a meal. It is then they are noticed and prompt treatment to destroy them is advised. Remove and launder the pet's bedding and use a pyrethrin-based airborne insecticide to treat the bed and rooms where fleas are seen. Vacuum floors to pick up dead and paralyzed fleas and use the cleaner's crevice tool to pick up lint and dust along baseboards. Discard the contents of the vacuum cleaner bag immediately. If the fleas reappear, repeat the treatment.

Common sense is the best precaution when using any insecticide. This includes reading the label prior to each use. Always wash hands after using and especially before eating or smoking. Select the right product for the job to be done and do not waste the product by using more than recommended on the label.

When outdoor insects are a problem, plants should be treated with multi-purpose House and Garden Bug Killer (or an equivalent product) about once a week and immediately after each rain. If the insect infestation is heavy, use the insecticide twice a week. Continue application as long as any insects remain in evidence. Be sure to apply product to the underside as well as the top of the leaves.

Appendix G

Keep liquid insecticides in their own containers until ready to use them. If a hand pump sprayer must be emptied for any reason once it has been filled with a liquid product, either dispose of the product or transfer it back to its original container. Insecticides should never be put into any container where they might be mistaken for food or other household products. Indoor spraying for flies is most effective at the brightest time of day. When light is dull, they tend to doze on walls and ceilings, but they buzz around and become active in bright light. They are hard to swat at this time, but are natural sponges for an airborne insecticide.

Surface insecticides

Insects play an important role in the ecological plan, but they become pests when they invade our living quarters. Many are known disease carriers and some species bite or sting. So in the home, it is important to get rid of insects such as cockroaches, ants and other types of crawling bugs as soon as they are discovered. Surface insecticides, sometimes called residual insecticides, are the best choice for control of crawing insect pests. They are applied to surfaces in the home where insects are likely to crawl. Dispensed as a coarse, wet spray, they dry quickly leaving a very thin deposit of insecticide on the treated surface. Their powerful ingredients remain active up to several weeks to kill insects long after the area has been treated. As insects crawl over treated areas, the insecticide is picked up and absorbed by their bodies, causing them to die. The ingredients in surface insecticides are not as fast-acting as those in airborne products, but they are effective for a longer time. Residual insecticides should never be sprayed into the air in the same manner as airborne insecticides. They are only applied to surfaces where bugs crawl.

Special tips

When insects invade the pantry, discard all infested foods. Cereal foods like crackers, cornmeal and prepared mixes are favorite targets and each container should be inspected for contamination. Remove all items from cupboards and if possible, wash shelves and walls with a disinfectant cleaning solution. After cleaning, treat cupboard corners and seams with a residual insecticide. Apply product where bugs can hide—in cracks and crevices, joints and where edges meet. Avoid contamination of foods, dishes, and cooking utensils by covering them or moving them away from the area where insecticide is being used. When

Insecticides

the insecticide has dried, line treated shelves and drawers with paper. Items can then be returned to storage and doors or drawers left ajar to dispel any noticeable odor.

Asphalt tile, plastic and rubber items may be sensitive to some of the ingredients in many insecticides. For this reason avoid excessive wetting when using on or near items made of these materials.

Spray window and door screens with a residual insecticide. This will discourage tiny pests like sand flies, midges and leafhoppers which can squeeze through the small openings in screens.

Sowbugs, centipedes and millipedes may be a problem in basements. Such insects hide in moist, dark areas and feed on rotting vegetation. They can enter the home through small cracks in the foundation or through basement windows. The first step in ridding the house of such pests is to check the foundation and repair any cracks or crevices. Then use a residual insecticide to treat surfaces where insects are seen crawling. However, avoid spraying on shrubbery or flowers. If there are plants near the foundation, keep these areas free of dried leaves, rotting vegetation and excessive moisture. Try to plant shrubs and flowers far enough away from the foundation so sunlight and wind can penetrate between them and the house. Clean shrubbery means fewer pests.

Most insecticides can be used around food preparation areas if a few simple precautions are followed. Always cover any exposed food and cooking utensils. If eating or cooking utensils have been left uncovered, wash in hot water with detergent before using them and discard any exposed food. . . .

Always store insecticides safely. Choose an area that is located away from heat sources and out of children's reach. Never transfer an insecticide from its own package into another container. It could be used incorrectly if the package directions are discarded, or it might be mistaken for food or another household product.

If ants are a problem in the home, try to determine what might be attracting them and learn where they are finding an entrance. First check for food spills and clean these away, then try to locate crawl paths and the ants' nest. Check the outside of the home for any cracks or crevices that may serve as entry points for the insects and treat these, the nest and crawl paths, with a residual insecticide. If the exact point of entry, crawl paths or

255

nest cannot be located, treat such areas as baseboards, moldings, window and door frames in rooms where the ants are seen.

Wood for the fireplace may bring unwanted insect pests into the home. If wood will be stored near the house, in the garage or indoors, treat the storage areas with a heavy-wetting dose of . . . insecticide before the wood is delivered and stacked. Repeat treatment around the edges of stacked wood at 6 week intervals.

Unseen hideouts can harbor roaches, water bugs, moths, carpet beetles, spiders, centipedes and silverfish. Check under heavy furnishings which sit directly on the floor and clean behind them so dust and lint does not accumulate. Also, clean behind cabinets not flush with walls. Periodically, treat crevices and corners with residual insecticide.

Stacks of lumber and discarded items in the yard are good hiding and breeding places for many kinds of insects. Keep the premises free of unwanted debris and clear away leaves and trash from window wells and the foundation—especially in the fall and spring. Also, keep basement and storage areas dry and free of unwanted items.

All insecticides have an EPA number listed on the container. This indicates that the product has been approved for use according to guidelines established by the Environmental Protection Agency (EPA) of the United States Government.

Eating and smoking are taboo when using insecticides. After using and storing these products, wash hands before eating or smoking. If insecticide spills on clothes, remove clothing and wash skin with soap and water. Garments should be laundered before wearing them again.

Entomologists say that most spiders are not really harmful, they are just annoying. In fact, they might be considered beneficial because they feed on small insects. Spiders are not really insects, but if they become a problem in the home, a residual insecticide can be used to control them. Webs and egg sacs should be removed and destroyed.

Direct spraying of an occasional insect will usually produce quick results. However, it may take a minute or two for some insects to react. Don't "drown" the insect and try to avoid spraying background surfaces or objects ... which might be damaged by the spray mist.

Be sure to choose the right product for the job to be done and to use insecticides according to their label directions. Product use directions have been carefully written to give as much information about the product and its use as possible. Also, products differ from each other and recommendations for use may vary from one product to another. Each time an insecticide is used, read the label again to be sure of good results.

Keep waste containers tightly covered and empty them often. If a food disposal unit is used, operate it after each meal. Rinse bottles, cans and jars before discarding them. Plastic bags or liners keep the interiors of containers clean, but they should still be washed occasionally and may be treated with a residual insecticide to keep insects away.

Safety tips for aerosol containers

- Be sure spray is aimed away from face.
- Avoid spraying while smoking or close to a fire or flame.
- Store where container is out of children's reach.
- Store where temperature will not reach or exceed 120 degrees F. (49 degrees C).
- Dispose of empty containers safely; do not puncture the container, incinerate it or throw it into any fire.

Appendix H
Emergency Treatment for Insecticide Poisoning

- Salvage the insecticide container. Antidotes and first-aid instructions are on the label.
- Remove the victim at once from the contaminated area.
- Remove contaminated clothing. Wash contaminated body areas with soap and water.
- Rush to the nearest medical aid.
- Institute artificial respiration if needed.
- Do not induce vomiting in a stuporous or unconscious victim.

Symptoms of severe organophosphate poisoning may be as follows:

Nausea and vomiting
Changes in heart rate
Muscle weakness
Respiratory distress
Sweating
Headache and visual disturbance
Confusion
Convulsions or coma

Such symptoms may begin almost at once, or they may be delayed, sometimes for as long as twelve hours following exposure.

Symptoms of carbamate poisoning are as follows:

Light-headedness and blurring of vision
Nausea and vomiting
Malaise
Excessive sweating and salivation

Symptoms of chlorinated hydrocarbon poisoning are as follows:

Nausea
Weakness and lethargy
Limb jerking
Confusion
Loss of appetite
Semiconsciousness

258

Appendix I
Nontoxic Homemade
Insecticides and Repellents

Garlic has been in use as a bug chaser since the early days of Egypt. Several sprays can be made that are effective against a number of garden pests such as aphids and mosquito larvae.

Recipe 1:
Blend 3 cloves of garlic, 1 chopped onion, and 2 cups of water. Add 2 teaspoons hot red pepper. Allow to steep for twenty-four hours, strain, dilute with 5 cups of water, and spray.

Recipe 2:
Blend 2 cloves of garlic, 3 hot peppers, 3 tablespoons of chopped chives, and 1½ cups of water. Let steep twenty-four hours, strain, add 1 tablespoon soap powder, dilute with 7 cups of water, and spray.

Other home remedies include pennyroyal leaves rubbed on the skin to ward off mosquitoes, and a wormwood-tea spray that is said to be effective against flies and fleas. A weak soap-and-water solution is supposed to get rid of soft-bodied insects. A teaspoon of mineral oil poured onto the ends of new corn will, it is said, prevent worms from getting into the ear.

Appendix J
Classification of Insects
Discussed in This Book

Kingdom: Animalia
Phylum: Arthropoda
    Class: Arachnida (arachnids). The Arachnida are mainly nonaquatic, possess 4 or 5 pairs of legs, breathe air, and have pincers or fangs rather than jaws and antennae. There are about 30,000 species in the class.
    Orders: Acarina (mites and ticks)
          Araneida (spiders)
          Scorpionida (scorpions)
    Class: Insecta (insects). Most Insecta breathe air and live on land. They possess three distinct body parts: head, thorax, and abdomen. Most possess two pairs of wings. There are about 700,000 species in the class.
    Orders: Anaplura (lice)—*anoplos*, unarmed; *oura*, tail
          Blattaria (cockroaches)—*blatta*, insect that shuns light
          Coleoptera (beetles)—*coleos*, sheath; *ptera*, wings
          Diptera (flies)—*dis*, two; *ptera*, wings
          Ephemeroptera (mayflies)—*ephemeros*, living but a day
          Hemiptera (bugs)—*hemi*, half; *ptera*, wings
          Hymenoptera (bees)—*hymen*, membrane; *ptera*, wings
          Lepidoptera (moths, butterflies)—*lepidos*, scale; *ptera*, wings
          Siphonaptera (fleas)—*siphon*, tube; *aptera*, wingless
          Thysanoptera (thrips)—*thysanos*, frings; *ptera*, wings

Classifications of Insects

Trichoptera (caddis flies)—*thrix,* hair; *ptera,* wings

Class: Chilopoda (centipedes). The Chilopoda have anywhere from 15 to 173 body segments with a pair of jointed appendages on each segment. There are about 2,000 species.

Appendix K
Delusions of Parasitosis

It should be noted that the very idea of insect infestation of the body and head can be a symptom of profound emotional disturbance or of mental illness. Such patients are very difficult for the physician to handle, whether he is an allergist, a dermatologist, or a general practitioner. They are not easily argued out of the delusion that they are being overrun by "bugs." They will scratch themselves raw, pick at their skin until wounds cannot heal, and often develop secondary infection of some magnitude. It is difficult to convince them when tests show no organic cause for their itching and no parasites can be found. Such patients have been classified into four categories: those who suffer from a toxic psychosis, such as that which occurs as a result of alcoholism, pellagra, some medications, or prolonged fever; those who are schizophrenic; those with involutional melancholia; and those suffering from paranoia. Toxic psychosis is naturally approached by treating the underlying physical problem that is causing the delusion. The delusion of infestation by "bugs" among the schizophrenic is usually a relatively minor symptom in the over-all picture of disturbed behavior. The delusion of parasitosis among those in the third and fourth groups, however, presents real difficulties for the physician. Their delusion is very real, and getting them to psychiatric help is often very difficult. The physician is uncomfortably aware that those suffering from involutional melancholia may well be suicidal; while those who are paranoid may be dangerous to others as well as to themselves.

Symptoms of this strange delusion are diagnosed first by ruling out organic causes for itching skin and then by ruling out the presence of any insect parasites such as mites or fleas. Once it is clear that the patient is delusional, he will need superhuman patience and understanding.

Books of Interest

Bandsma, Arend T., and Rolin T. Brandt. *The Amazing World of Insects*. New York: Macmillan Company, 1963.

Dethier, Vincent G. *To Know a Fly*. San Francisco: Holden-Day Inc., 1962.

_____. *The Physiology of Insect Senses*. New York: John Wiley & Sons, Inc., 1963.

Fox, Richard M., and Jean Walker Fox. *Introduction to Comparative Entomology*. New York: Reinhold Publishing Company, 1964.

Frazier, Claude A., M.D. *Insect Allergy*. St. Louis: Warren H. Green, Inc., 1969.

Grout, Roy A. *The Hive and the Honey Bee*. Hamilton, Ill.: Dadant & Sons, 1946.

Headstrom, Richard. *Nature in Miniature*. New York: Alfred A. Knopf, 1968.

Lehane, Brendan. *The Compleat Flea*. New York: The Viking Press, 1969.

Nachtigoll, Werner. *Insects in Flight*. New York: McGraw-Hill Book Co., 1968.

Zinsser, Hans. *Rats, Lice, and History*. Boston: Little, Brown & Company, Inc., 1934.

Index

Acarina: *see* mites and ticks
Allergens: 17–8
"Allergic load": 19–20, 21
Allergic reactions: 16–21, 23, 51–52, 56–58, 60–62, 95–97, 112, 191, 196, 241–42; factors in, 18–19; symptoms of, 52, 57–58, 95–97, 241; treatment of, 60–62, 241–42
Allergy: 14–23, 53–56, 59–60, 241–42; definition of, 16, 23; incidence of, 16, 18, 59–60; mechanism of, 16–17; role of heredity, 17; sensitization in, 17–18, 20–21, 96, 196; factors in, 18–20, 23; multiple allergies, 19, 23, 59–60; characteristics of the insect allergic, 21–22; skin tests, 21, 53–54;

diagnosis, 55–56; *see also* avoidance of stinging insects
American trypanosomiasis: *see* sleeping sickness
Anaphylactic shock: 16, 19, 52, 56, 58, 97, 112–13, 191, 196, 241–42; to honeybees, 16, 56; symptoms, 52, 58, 241; from mosquitoes, 97; from blackflies, 112–13; from bedbugs, 191; from kissing bugs, 196; treatment, 241–42
Anophelinae: *see* mosquitoes
Ants: 10, 12, 39, 78–88, 231; number of species, 78; ecology, 79–82; red harvester, 39, 83, 86; fire ant, 10, 39, 83–88, 231

Index